TEST YOUR PHYSICAL FITNESS

TEST YOUR PHYSICAL FITNESS

DR. C. ASHOK

KALPAZ

Published by

Kalpaz Publications
C-30, Satyawati Nagar,
Delhi – 110052
Ph.: 011-47034999, 9811692060
www.kalpazpublications.com
E-mail: kalpaz@hotmail.com

Distribution Network
gyanbooks.com
India, USA, Canada, UK, Australia, France

ISBN: 978-81-7835-681-5 (HB)

Reprint in India, 2024
First Published, 2008

Printed at: Gyan Press, Delhi.

Test Your Physical Fitness
Author: Dr. C. Ashok

Dedicated to
My Dear Friend
A.Ramasubramanian @ Mani @ Pulavar
S/O Athimoolam (Guarder)
Physical Education Teacher,
Manal Vinayagar Koil Street,
Settur – Rajapalayam.

Contents

List of Tables

List of Figures

Preface

The book "*Test Your Physical Fitness*" is my third issue that shall assist the research scholars in the field of Physical Education and Sports Sciences in general and persons longing for knowing their level of physical fitness in particular. It is a compendium of physical fitness testing procedures. I tried my level best to list out the testing procedures in the field of Physical Education and Sports Sciences with which a researcher or tester can definitely achieve his or her goal. This book is a resultant outcome of my difficulties faced during my research and I hope that the younger generation may not face the same in testing variables during their research. I sincerely express my gratitude to our Correspondent and Principal for having positively shown gesture in my career and with out their magnanimity, this book would not have been formulated. All the suggestions and criticisms are welcomed.

C. Ashok

1

1-RM Tests (Repetition maximum tests)

Purpose: to measure maximum strength of various muscle and muscle groups.

Description / procedure: One repetition maximum tests (1-RM) is a popular method of measuring isotonic muscle strength. It is a measure of the maximal weight a subject can lift with one repetition. It is important to reach the maximum weight without prior fatiguing the muscles. After a warm up, choose a weight that is achievable. Then after a rest of at least several minutes, increase the weight and try again. The athletes chooses subsequent weights until they can only repeat one full and correct lift of that weight.

Scoring: the maximum weight lifted is recorded. The sequence of lifts should also be recorded as these can be used in subsequent tests to help in determining the lifts to attempt. To standardize the score it may be useful to calculate a score proportional to the person's bodyweight.

Equipment required: Free weights (barbells, dumbbells) or other gym equipment.

Advantages: the required equipment is readily available in most gymnasiums.

Disadvantages: performing a maximum weight lift is only for advances weight trainers. It is important to have good technique before attempting this test.

Comments: The test results will be specific to the equipment used and the technique allowed, so is best used for test-retest measures. The test is also called one rep max, 1-RM, one repetition maximum

Variations / modifications: Sometimes a three or five repetition maximum is used, particularly for less experienced lifters. These greater reps would require less weight and may be considered less dangerous. Changing the number of repetition also changes the muscle energy systems and validity of this test.

2

1 Mile Walk Test

Description: The purpose of this test is to walk as fast as possible for 1 mile. After you have completed the mile, immediately take your pulse rate. If you do not have a heart rate monitor, you can manually count the number of beats for 10 seconds, and then multiply that by 6 to get your minute heart rate. Note the time it took to complete the mile.
Scoring: A VO_{2max} score can be calculated using the following equation:
females: VO_2 = 139.168 - (0.388 x age) - (0.077 x weight in lb.) - (3.265 x walk time in minutes) - (0.156 x heart rate).
males: add 6.318 to the equation for females above.
Equipment required: stopwatch, smooth and level marked 1 mile track, paper and pencil, heart rate monitor (optional).
Target population: Suitable for both males and females of poor fitness who would not be able to complete a similar distance run test.
Advantages: minimal equipment and costs are required, and the test can be self-administered.
Disadvantages: This test is too easy for highly fit people. Also, since you must walk as fast as possible, the accuracy of this test depends on your pacing ability and level of motivation.

3

1-RM Bench Press

Purpose: to measure maximum strength of the chest muscle groups.
Equipment required: Bench with safety, bar and various free weights.
Description / procedure: The subject should perform an adequate warmup. An example would be to warm up with 5-10 reps of a light-to-moderate weight, then after a minute rest perform two heavier warm-up sets of 2-5 reps, with a two-minute rest between sets. The subject should then rest two to four minutes, then perform the one-rep-max attempt with proper technique. If the lift is successful, rest for another two to four minutes and increase the load 5-10%, and attempt another lift. If the subject fails to perform the lift with correct technique, rest two to four minutes and attempt a weight 2.5-5% lower. Keep increasing and decreasing the weight until a maximum left is performed. Selection of the starting weight is crucial so that the maximum lift is completed within approximately five attempts after the warm-up sets.
Scoring: the maximum weight lifted is recorded. To standardize the score it may be useful to calculate a score proportional to the person's bodyweight. The sequence of lifts should also be recorded as these can be used in subsequent

Table - 1

1 Rep Max Bench Press Table for adults (weight lifted per bodyweight)

Rating	*Score (per body weight)*
Excellent	> 1.60
Good	1.30 - 1.60
Average	1.15 - 1.29
Below Average	1.00 - 1.14
Poor	0.91 - 0.99
Very Poor	< 0.90

tests to help in determining the starting lifts. See the table below for general guidelines for interpreting the results, based on my personal experiences.

Equipment required: Bench with safety, bar and free weights (including light weights).

Advantages: the required equipment is readily available in most gymnasiums, and the test is simple to perform

Disadvantages: This test should only be performed by those experienced at performing the bench press lift with good technique. Good technique will also enable the lifter to maximize their score.

Comments: For safety, a spotter should stand at the head of the bench throughout the test. The results of this test may be specific to the equipment used (height of bench, variations in weights), so is best to use the same equipment for test-retest measures. The warm up procedure should also be recorded and repeated with further testing. If any variation in technique was allowed, this should be recorded on the results sheet for referral when the test is repeated. The test is also called one rep max, 1-RM, and one repetition maximum.

Variations / modifications: Sometimes a three or five repetition maximum is used, particularly for less experienced lifters. These greater reps would require less weight and may be considered less dangerous. Changing the number of repetition also changes the muscle energy systems and validity of this test.

This test forms part of the Navy Physical Readiness Test (PRT), performed by US Navy personnel every six months. An alternative to this test is the 500 yard swim test.

Purpose: This test measures aerobic fitness and leg muscles endurance.

Equipment required: 1.5 mile flat and hard running course, stopwatch

Description / procedure: The aim of this test is to complete the 1.5 mile course in the shortest possible time. At the start, all soldiers line up behind the starting line. On the command 'go,' the clock will start, and you will begin running at your own pace. Although walking is authorized, it is strongly discouraged. A cool down walk should be performed at the completion of the test.

Scoring: The total time to complete the course is recorded.

Comments: It is permitted to pace a participant (such as running ahead of, along side of, or behind) during the run, as long as there is no physical contact with the runner and it does not physically hinder other people taking the test. Cheering or calling out the elapsed time is also permitted. During the 1.5-mile run, it is critical to have some type of medical support in place or a medical emergency plan, Dangerous climate conditions such as hot/humid weather should be avoided and water or other fluids should be made available upon completion of the assessment.

4

10 and 30-second Tri-level Anaerobic Tests

Equipment required: Repco front access cycle ergometer (which uses air resistance to modify workload), work monitor unit, stopwatch, scales to record subjects mass.

Description / procedure: The subject is instructed to pedal as fast as possible for 10 or 30 seconds. The feet must the firmly strapped onto the pedal to enable maximal power output. Strong verbal encouragement will help the subject achieve their maximal score. For the 10 second test, you may want to give the athlete two attempts, with five minutes break between, and record the best effort. Latest model recording units can record power and work output every second, with older units work output can be recorded manually at selected time intervals.

Scoring: The measurements that can be gained from the work monitor unit are total work (Alactic Work Index) and peak power (Alactic Power Index), and for the 30 second test (Lactic Work Index) a fatigue index can be calculated from the decline in power throughout the test. Peak power and total work scores can be divided by body weight for relative scores, and norm tables are available for these tests.

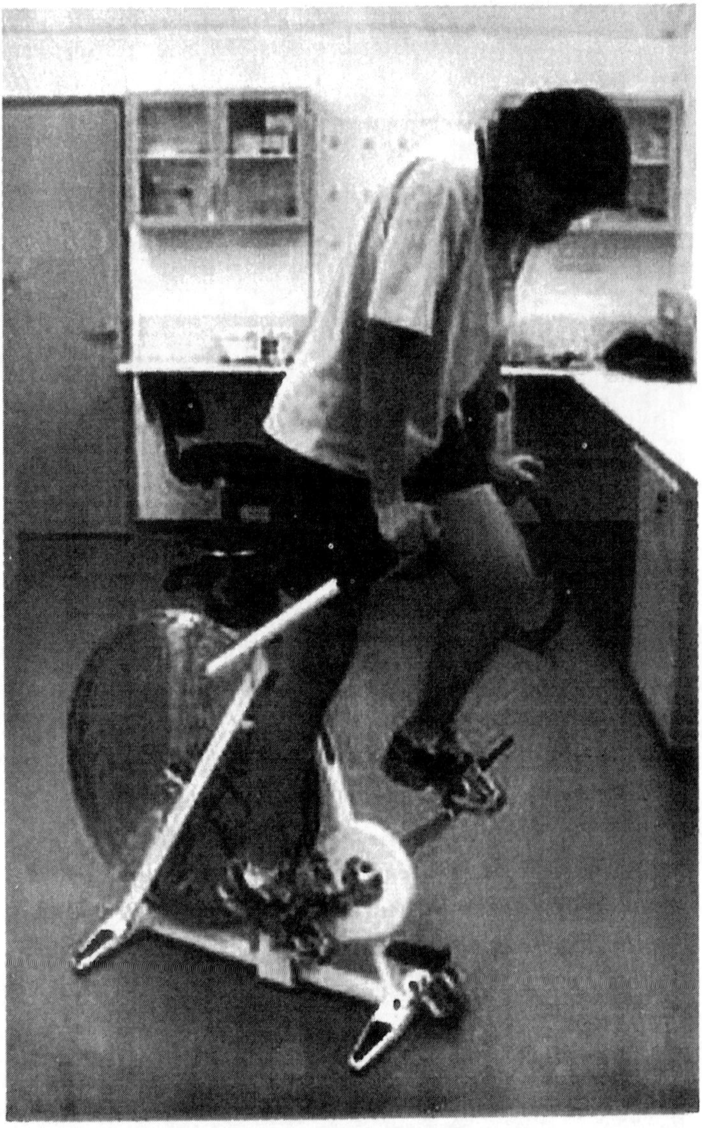

Fig. 1. Cycle Engometer

5

150 Metre Endurance Test

Objective

To monitor the development of the athlete's endurance for the 100 metres event.

Required Resources

To undertake this test you will require:

400 metre track - 150 metre marked section

Stop watch

Assistant

How to conduct the test

The test comprises of a 150 metre run from a standing start. The assistant records the time for the athlete to complete 150 metres.

6

Beep

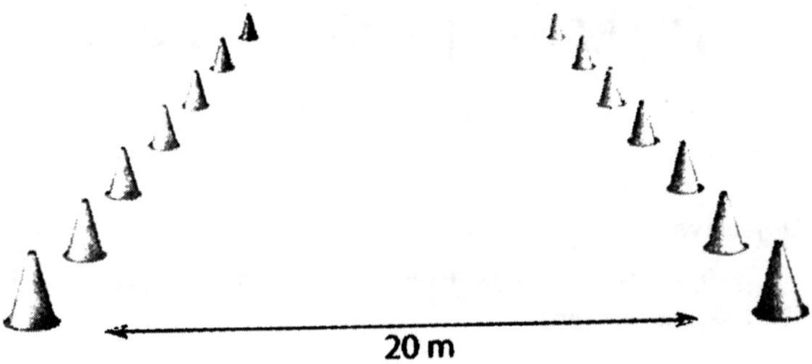

Fig. 2. Marking Cones-1

Equipment required: Flat, non-slip surface, marking cones, 20m measuring tape, pre-recorded audio tape, tape recorder, recording sheets.

Description: This test involves continuous running between two lines 20m apart in time to recorded beeps. For this reason the test if also often called the 'beep' or 'bleep' test. The time between recorded beeps decrease each minute (level). There are several versions of the test, but one commonly used version has an initial running velocity of 8.5 km/hr, which increases by 0.5 km/hr each minute (more on test variations).

Scoring: The athletes score is the level and number of shuttles reached before they were unable to keep up with the tape recording. This score can be converted to a VO2max equivalent score using this calculator.

- **Target population:** Suitable for sports teams and school groups, but not for populations in which a maximal exercise test would be contraindicated.
- **Validity:** There are published VO_{2max} score equivalents for each level reached (calculator available here). The correlation to actual VO_{2max} scores is high.
- **Reliability:** Reliability would depend on how strictly the test is run, and the practice allowed for the subjects.
- **Advantages:** Large groups can perform this test all at once for minimal costs. Also, the test continues to maximum effort unlike many other tests of endurance capacity.
- **Disadvantages:** Practice and motivation levels can influence the score attained, and the scoring can be subjective. As the test is usually conducted outside, the environmental conditions can be often affect the results.

Other considerations:

- As the audio-tapes may stretch over time, the tapes need to be calibrated which involves timing a one-minute interval and making adjustment to the distance between markers. The recording is also available on compact disc, which does not require such a stringent calibration, but should also be checked occasionally
- This test goes by many names, though you need to be careful as the different names also may signify that these are different versions of the test. Therefore you need to be wary when comparing results or comparing to norms.
- This test is a maximal test, which requires a reasonable level of fitness. It is not recommended for recreational athletes or people with health problems, injuries or low fitness levels.

7

Sit and Reach Test

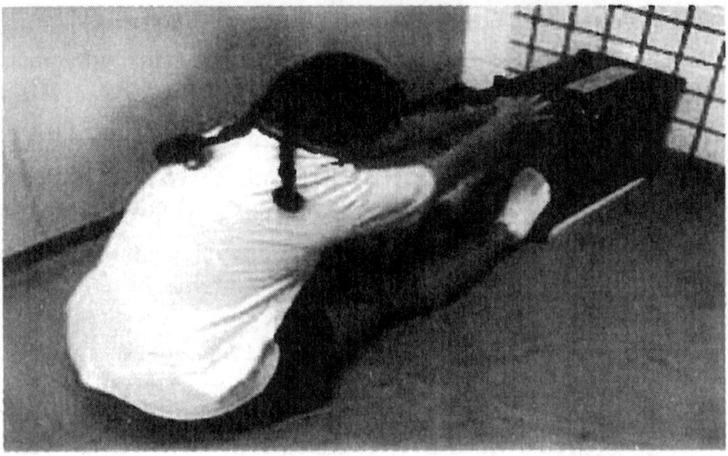

Fig. 3. Sit and Reach.

This test measures the flexibility of the lower back and hamstring muscles. This following describes the procedures as used in the President's Challenge Fitness Awards.

Description / procedure: This test involves sitting on the floor with legs out straight ahead. Feet (shoes off) are placed with the soles flat against the box, shoulder-width apart. Both knees are held flat against the floor by the tester. With hands on top of each other and palms facing down, the subject reaches forward along the measuring line as far as possible. After three practice reaches, the fourth reach is held for at least two seconds while the distance is recorded. Make sure there is no jerky movements, and that the fingertips remain level and the legs flat.

Scoring: The score is recorded to the nearest centimeter as the distance before (negative) or beyond (positive) the toes. The procedures for the Presidents Challenge require that the box is made with 23 centimeters at the level of the feet, so 10 cm past the toes is recorded as 33 cm. The table below gives you a guide for expected scores (in cm) for adults using zero at the level of the feet (add 23 if using the other method).

Table 2. Sit and Reach Score

	Men	*Women*
super	> +27	> +30
excellent	+17 to +27	+21 to +30
good	+6 to +16	+11 to +20
average	0 to +5	+1 to +10
fair	-8 to -1	-7 to 0
poor	-19 to -9	-14 to -8
very poor	< -20	< -15

Equipment required: sit and reach box (or alternatively a ruler can be used, and held between the feet).

Validity: This tests only measures the flexibility of the lower back and hamstrings, and is a valid measure of this.

Reliability: The reliability will depends on the amount of warm-up allowed, and whether the same procedures are followed each time. Most norms are based on no previous warm-up, though the best results will be achieved after a warm up or if the test is proceeded by a test such as the endurance test.

Advantages: This is the most commonly used test of flexibility, so there is lots of data for comparison. Also, it is a easy and quick test to perform.

Disadvantages: Variations in arm, leg and trunk length can make comparisons between individuals misleading. The best measures are made with a measurement box specifically made for this test, which is not readily available. This test is specific to the range of motion and muscles and joints of the lower back and hamstrings.

Other comments: Lower back flexibility is important because tightness in this area is implicated in lumbar lordosis, forward pelvic tilt and lower back pain.

8

Handgrip Strength Test

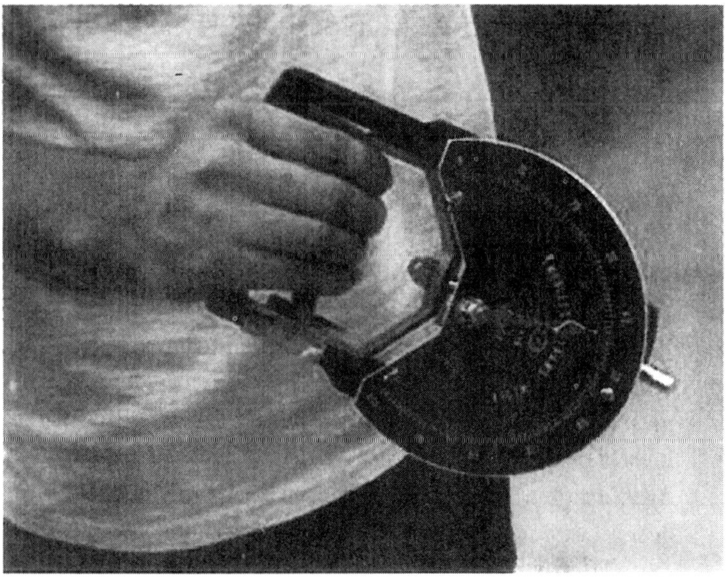

Fig. 4. Handgrip Dynamometer

The purpose of this test is to measure grip or forearm muscle strength. Handgrip strength is important for any sport in which the hands are used for catching, throwing or lifting. Also, as a general rule people with strong hands tend to be strong elsewhere.

Equipment required: handgrip dynamometer

Description / procedure: The subject to be tested holds the dynamometer in one hand in line with the forearm and hanging by the thigh. Maximum grip strength is then determined without swinging the arm.

- **Scoring:** The best of two trials for each hand is recorded. The values listed below (in kilograms) give a guide to expected scores for adults. They are the average of the best scores of each hand.

Table 3. Handgrip Strength

*Rating**	*Males (kg)*	*Females (kg)*
excellent	> 64	> 38
very good	56-64	34-38
above average	52-56	30-34
average	48-52	26-30
below average	44-48	22-26
poor	40-44	20-22
very poor	< 40	< 20

* Source and population group unknown.

- **Validity:** The validity of this test as a measure of general strength has been questioned, as the strength of the forearm muscles does not necessarily represent the strength of other muscle groups.
- **Advantages:** This is a simple and commonly used test of general strength level.
- **Disadvantages:** The dynamometer must be adjusted for hand size, how successfully this is done will affect the accuracy of the measurement.
- **Comments:** It is also useful to record whether the athlete is left or right handed, as this may help in the interpretation of results. The non-dominant hand usually scores about 10% lower.

9

Vertical Jump Test (Sargent Jump)

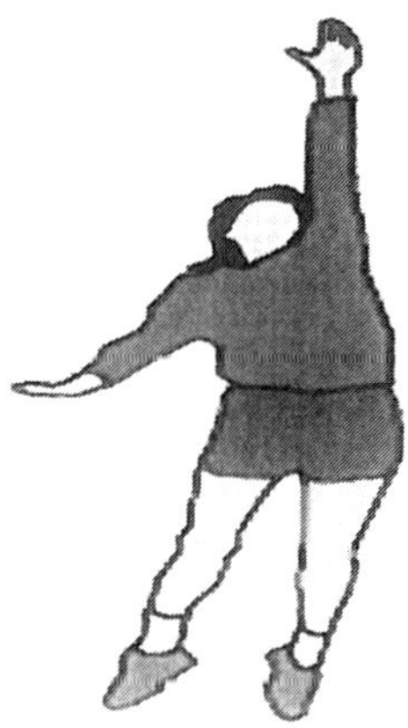

Fig. 5. Sargent Jump

This procedure describes the method used for directly measuring the height jumped. There are also timing systems that measure the time of the jump and from that calculate the jump height.

Equipment required: measuring tape or marked wall, chalk for marking wall and jump mat.

Description / procedure (see also variations below): the athlete stands side on to a wall and reaches up with the hand closest to the wall. Keeping the feet flat on the ground, the point of the fingertips is marked or recorded. This is called the standing reach. The athlete then stands away from the wall, and jumps vertically as high as possible using both arms and legs to assist in projecting the body upwards. Attempt to touch the wall at the highest point of the jump. The difference in distance between the standing reach height and the jump height is the score. The best of three attempts is recorded.

Variations: The vertical jump test can also be performed using a specialized apparatus called the Vertec. The procedure when using the Vertec is very similar to as described above. Jump height can also be measured using a jump mat which measures the displacement of the hips. To be accurate, you must ensure the feet land back on the mat with legs nearly fully extended. Vertical jump height can also be measured using a timing mat. The vertical jump test is usually performed with a counter movement, where there is bending of the knees prior to the jump. The test can also be performed as a squat jump, starting from the position of knees being bent. Other test variations are to perform the test with no arm movement (one hand on hip, the other raised above the head) to isolate the leg muscles and reduce the effect of variations in coordination of the arm movements. The test can also be performed off one leg, with a step into the jump, or with a run-up, depending on the relevance to the sport involved.

Scoring: The jump height Jump is usually recorded as the score in distance. The table below provides a ranking scale for adult athletes based on my observations, and will give a general idea of what is a good score. For more information, see a selection of vertical jump test results.

There are also a calculation to convert jump height into a power or work score. Here are several formula I have come across.

Power = 2.21 x weight x root of jump distance.

Power = body mass(kg) x (4.9 x height jumped in meters)^2

Peak Anaerobic Power output (Watts)

PAPw = (60.7 x jump height) + (45.3 x body mass(kg) - 2055 (ref: Sayers et al.)

Advantages: this test is simple and quick to perform.

Table 4. Sargent Jump

Rating	*Males (inches)*	*Males (cm)*	*Females (inches)*	*Females (cm)*
excellent	> 28	> 70	> 24	> 60
very good	24 - 28	61-70	20 - 24	51-60
above average	20 - 24	51-60	16 - 20	41-50
average	16 - 20	41-50	12 - 16	31-40
below average	12 - 16	31-40	8 - 12	21-30
poor	8 - 12	21-30	4 - 8	11-20
very poor	< 8	< 21	< 4	< 11

Disadvantages: technique plays a part in maximizing your score, as the subject must time the jump so that the wall is marked at the peak of the jump.

Comments: The jump height can be affected by how much you bend your knees before you jump, and the effective use of the arms. The test is also sometimes incorrectly spelled as the "Sergeant" or "Sargent" Test.

History: This method described above for measuring a person's vertical jump height is sometimes known as a Sargent Jump, named after Dudley Sargent, who was one of the pioneers in American physical education.

10

Fitness Testing

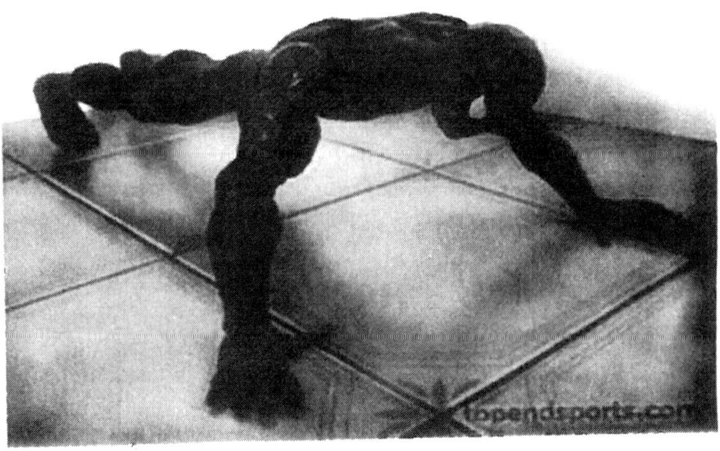

Fig. 6. Push Up

Push Up Test

How many can you do? Men should use the standard "military style" pushup position with only the hands and the toes touching the floor. Women have the additional option of using the "bent knee" position. To do this, kneel on the floor, hands on either side of the chest and keep your back straight. Do as many push ups as possible until exhaustion. Count the total number of pushups performed. Use the chart below to find out how you rate.

Table 5. Push Up Test (Men)

Age	*17-19*	*20-29*	*30-39*	*40-49*	*50-59*	*60-65*
Excellent	>56	>47	>41	>34	>31	>30
Good	47-56	39-47	34-41	28-34	25-31	24-30
Above average	35-46	30-39	25-33	21-28	18-24	17-23
Average	19-34	17-29	13-24	11-20	9-17	6-16
Below average	11-18	10-16	8-12	6-10	5-8	3-5
Poor	4-10	4-9	2-7	1-5	1-4	1-2
Very Poor	<4	<4	<2	0	0	0

Table 6. Push Up Test (Women)

Age	*17-19*	*20-29*	*30-39*	*40-49*	*50-59*	*60-65*
Excellent	>35	>36	>37	>31	>25	>23
Good	27-35	30-36	30-37	25-31	21-25	19-23
Above Average	21-27	23-29	22-30	13-24	15-20	13-18
Average	11-20	12-22	10-21	8-17	7-14	5-12
Below average	6-10	7-11	5-9	4-7	3-6	2-4
Poor	2-5	2-6	1-4	1-3	1-2	1
Very Poor	0-1	0-1	0	0	0	0

11

Illinois Agility Test

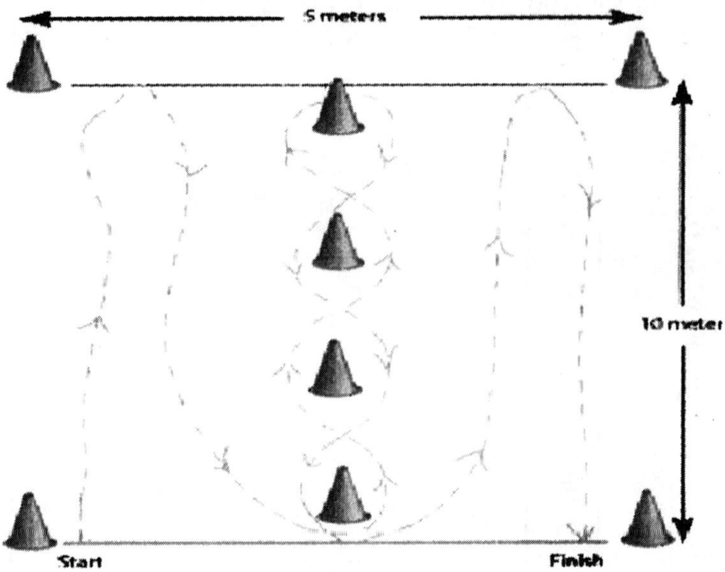

Fig. 7. Marking Cones - 2

Purpose: Agility is an important component of many team sports

Equipment required: flat non-slip surface, marking cones, stopwatch, measuring tape, timing gates (optional)

Description: The length of the course is 10 meters and the width (distance between the start and finish points) is 5 meters. Four cones are used to mark the start, finish and the two turning points. Another four cones are placed down the center an equal distance apart. Each cone in the center is spaced 3.3 meters apart.

Procedure: Subjects should lie on their front (head to the start line) and hands by their shoulders. On the 'Go' command the stopwatch is started, and the athlete gets up as quickly as possible and runs around the course in the direction indicated, without knocking the cones over, to the finish line, at which the timing is stopped.

Results: The table below gives some rating scores for the test

Table 7. Agility Run Ratings

Rating	*Males*	*Females*
Excellent	<15.2	<17.0
Good	16.1-15.2	17.9-17.0
Average	18.1-16.2	21.7-18.0
Fair	18.3-18.2	23.0-21.8
Poor	>18.3	>23.0

Advantages: This is a simple test to administer, requiring little equipment. Can test players ability to turn in different directions, and different angles.

Disadvantages: Choice of footwear and surface of area can effect times greatly. Results can be subject to timing inconsistencies, which may be overcome by using timing gates. Cannot distinguish between left and right turning ability.

Variations: the starting and finishing sides can be swapped, so that turning direction is reversed.

12

Home Step Test

This test is designed to measure your cardiovascular endurance. Using a 12 inch high bench (or a similar sized stair in your house), step on and off for 3 minutes Step up with one foot and then the other. Step down with one foot followed by the other foot. Try to maintain a steady four beat cycle. It's easy to maintain if you say "up, up, down, down". Go at a steady and consistent pace. At the end of 3 minutes, remain standing while you immediately check your heart rate by taking your pulse for one minute. Go here for more information about taking your heart rate, and see also other step tests.

Results

Compare your result to the chart below. This home step test is based loosely on the Canadian Home Fitness Test and the results below are also based from data collected performing this test.

Table 8. 3 Minute Step Test (Men)

Age	*18-25*	*26-35*	*36-45*	*46-55*	*56-65*	*65+*
Excellent	<79	<81	<83	<87	<86	<88
Good	79-89	81-89	83-96	87-97	86-97	88-96
Above Average	90-99	90-99	97-103	98-105	98-103	97-103
Average	100-105	100-107	104-112	106-116	104-112	104-113
Below Average	106-116	108-117	113-119	117-122	113-120	114-120
Poor	117-128	118-128	120-130	123-132		

13

Cooper 12 Minute Run

- **Purpose:** to test aerobic fitness (the ability of the body to use oxygen to power it while running)
- **Equipment required:** flat oval or running track, marking cones, recording sheets, stop watch.
- **Description / procedure:** Place markers at set intervals around the track to aid in measuring the completed distance. Participants run for 12 minutes, and the distance covered is recorded. Walking is allowed, though the participants must be encouraged to push themselves as hard as they can.
- **Scoring:** There are several equations that can be used to estimate VO_{2max} (in ml/kg/min) from the distance score (a formula for either kms or miles):

The table below also gives general guidelines for interpreting the results of this test for adults. These results are based on a few sources and are only approximate values.

$$VO_{2max} = (35.97 \times \text{miles}) - 11.29.$$

$$VO_{2max} = (22.351 \times \text{kilometers}) - 11.288$$

- **Target population:** This test can be modified to be suitable for most populations. For those who are unfit or unable to run, there are similar walking tests that can be performed.

Table 9. Results for Adult Males

Rating	*Distance (Meters)*
excellent	> 2700 m
good	2300 - 2700 m
average	1900 - 2300 m
below average	1500 - 1900 m
poor	< 1500 m

- **Validity:** Cooper (1968) reported a correlation of 0.90 between VO2max and the distance covered in a 12 min walk/run.
- **Reliability:** the reliability of this test would depend on practice, pacing strategies and motivation level. There should be good reliability if these issues are addressed.
- **Advantages:** large groups can be tested at once, and it is a very cheap and simple test to perform.
- **Disadvantages:** practice and pacing is required, and performance on this test can be affected greatly by motivation.
- **Variations / modifications:** The test can also be conducted by running on a treadmill for 12 minutes, set to level 1 (1 percent) incline to mimic outdoor running. There are many variations of the walk / run test. A very similar test is the Balke 15 minute run.

14

APFT 2 - Mile Run Test

This test forms part of the Army Physical Fitness Test (APFT), performed by US Army personnel every six months.

- **Purpose:** This test measures aerobic fitness and leg muscles endurance.

  Equipment required: 2 mile flat running course, stopwatch

  Description / procedure: The aim of this test is to complete the 2-mile course in the shortest possible time. At the start, all soldiers line up behind the starting line. On the command 'go,' the clock will start, and you will begin running at your own pace. Although walking is authorized, it is strongly discouraged.

  Scoring: The total time to complete the course is recorded. The scoring depends on the sex and age of the participant. See APFT for more information about scoring.

Comments: It is permitted to pace a soldier (such as running ahead of, along side of, or behind) during the run, as long as there is no physical contact with the runner and it does not physically hinder other soldiers taking the test. Cheering or calling out the elapsed time is also permitted.

15

3 Hop Test

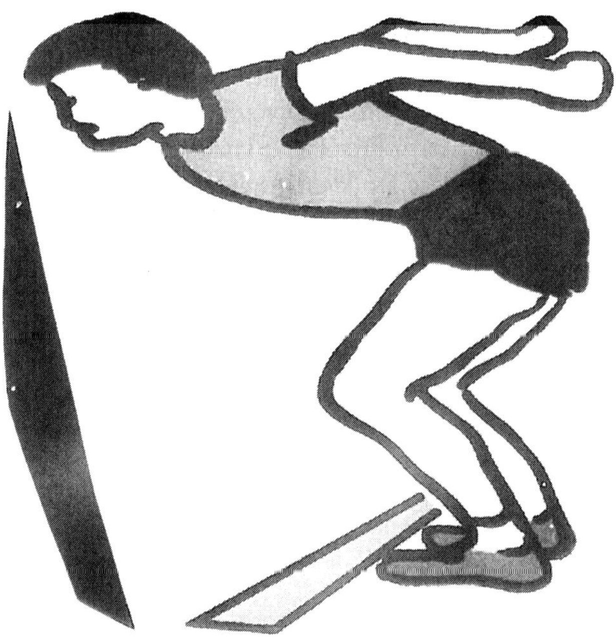

Fig. 8. Double Leg Hop

Purpose: to measure horizontal and vertical power of the legs with a component of balance and coordination.

Equipment required: tape measure to measure distance jumped, flat grass area. The starting take off line should be clearly marked.

Description / procedure: The aim of this test is to perform three consecutive double-leg hops as far as possible. Stretch out approximately 30 feet of rope or tape measure to mark the hopping direction and to aid recording the jump distance.The athlete starts by standing behind a line with feet shoulder width apart.When ready, they are to perform three consecutive broad jumps non-stop, using a forward as well as a vertical jump style that allows them to gain maximum distance. They are able to use their arms assist the explosive movement and for balance.

Scoring: The measurement is taken from take-off line to the nearest point of contact on the landing of the third jump (back of the heels). Record the longest distance jumped, the best of three trials.

Variations / modifications: A long jump landing pit may be used instead so that the final jump lands in the sand, which enables the subject to confidently put more effort into the final jump, and to extend the legs further in front of the body for landing. The test can also be conducted with any number of consecutive jumps.

Advantages: this test is simple and quick to perform, requiring minimal equipment.

Disadvantages: there is some skill component in this test.

Comments: Falling or stepping backward after the landing will result in measurement to that point of contact rather than where the feet first touched. Some subjects will try to use a step at take-off, which is not allowed.

16

20 Meter Shuttle Run Test

(alternate names: Multistage Fitness Test, MSFT, 20m Shuttle, Bleep Test)

The multistage fitness test, also known as the 20 meter shuttle run test, beep or bleep test among others, is nowadays a very common test of aerobic fitness.

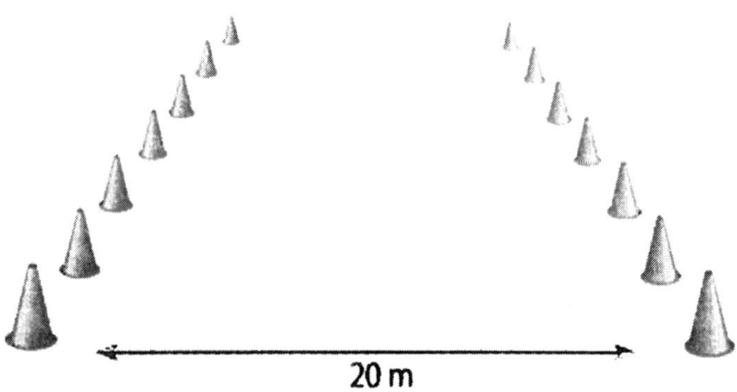

Fig. 9. Marking Cones - 1

Equipment required: Flat, non-slip surface, marking cones, 20m measuring tape, pre-recorded audio tape, tape recorder, recording sheets.

Description: This test involves continuous running between two lines 20m apart in time to recorded beeps. For this reason the test is also often called the 'beep' or 'bleep' test. The time between recorded beeps decrease each minute (level). There are several versions of the test, but one commonly used version has an initial running velocity of 8.5 km/hr, which increases by 0.5 km/hr each minute (more on test variations).

Scoring: The athletes score is the level and number of shuttles reached before they were unable to keep up with the tape recording. This score can be converted to a VO2max equivalent score using this calculator.

Target population: Suitable for sports teams and school groups, but not for populations in which a maximal exercise test would be contraindicated.

Validity: There are published VO_{2max} score equivalents for each level reached (calculator available here). The correlation to actual VO_{2max} scores is high.

Reliability: Reliability would depend on how strictly the test is run, and the practice allowed for the subjects.

Advantages: Large groups can perform this test all at once for minimal costs. Also, the test continues to maximum effort unlike many other tests of endurance capacity.

Disadvantages: Practice and motivation levels can influence the score attained, and the scoring can be subjective. As the test is usually conducted outside, the environmental conditions can be often affect the results.

Other considerations:

- As the audio-tapes may stretch over time, the tapes need to be calibrated which involves timing a one-minute interval and making adjustment to the distance between markers. The recording is also available on compact disc, which does not require such a stringent calibration, but should also be checked occasionally.
- This test goes by many names, though you need to be careful as the different names also may signify that these are different versions of the test. Therefore you need to be wary when comparing results or comparing to norms.

- This test is a maximal test, which requires a reasonable level of fitness. It is not recommended for recreational athletes or people with health problems, injuries or low fitness levels.

17

20 Yard Agility Test

This test is part of a battery for the USA Women's Soccer Team. The NFL use a very similar test for the NFL Combine Testing, the 20 yard shuttle.

- **Purpose:** The 20 yard agility run is a simple measure of an athlete's ability to accelerate, decelerate, change direction, and to accelerate again.

  Equipment required: start/stop timing gates or stopwatch, tape measure, non-slip running surface, cone markers.

  Description / procedure: Set up three marker cones in a straight line, exactly five yards apart - cones B, A (center) and C. At each cone place a line across using marking tape. The timer is positioned at the level of the center A cone, facing the athlete. The athlete straddles the center cone A with feet an equal distance apart and parallel to the line of cones. When ready, the athlete runs to cone B (touching the line with either foot), turns and accelerates to cone C (touching the line), and finishes by accelerating through the line at cone A. The stopwatch is started on the first movement of the athlete and stops the watch when the athlete's torso crosses the center line.

  Scoring: Record the best time of two trials.

  Comments: Encourage athletes to accelerate through the finish line to maximize their result.

18

30 - Second Wingate Test

Purpose: the aim of this test is to measure the anaeroic power of the lower body.
Equipment required: Fleisch or a modified Monark cycle ergometer.
Description / procedure: The subject should first perform a cycling warm up of several minutes. The subject is instructed to pedal as fast as possible for 30 seconds. In the first few seconds, the resistance load is adjusted to the pre-determined level, which is usually about 45 g/kg body weight (Fleisch) or 75 g/kg body weight (Monark) for adults. Power athletes would generally use high resistances, while children and older athletes may use lower.
Scoring: Some of the measures that can be gained from this test are mean and peak power (ideally measured in first five second interval of the test, expressed in watts (W)), relative peak power (determined by dividing peak power by body mass, expressed as W/kg) and a fatigue index determined from the decline in power.
Variations: an arm ergometer can also be used to measure upper body anaerobic power.
Comments: The Wingate test is also known as the Wingate Anaerobic Test (WANT), and was developed at the Wingate Institute in Israel during the 1970s.

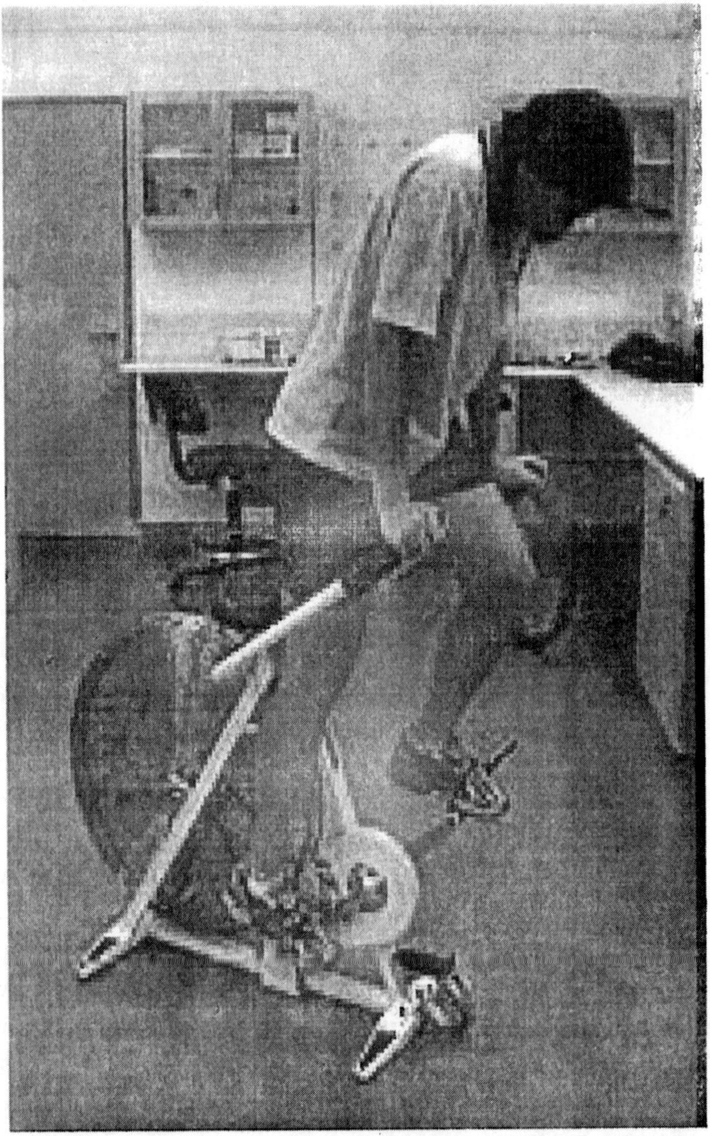

Fig. 10. Cycle Ergometer

19

90/90 Active Knee Extension (AKE) Hamstring Flexibility Test

Purpose: to assess the range of active knee extension in a position of hip flexion, as required in running and kicking.
Equipment required: goniometer with extended arms and spirit level (optional), and a firm table.
Description / procedure: The subject lies supine, head back and arms across the chest. The hip is passively flexed until the thigh is vertical (use the spirit level if available). Maintain this thigh position throughout the test, with the opposite leg in a fully extended position. The foot of the leg being tested is kept relaxed, while the leg is actively straightened until the point when the thigh begins to move from the vertical position. The thigh angle at this point is recorded.
Mmeasurement: measure the minimum angle of knee flexion with the thigh in the vertical position. The measurement unit is degrees. If the leg is able to be fully straightened, the angle would be recorded as 0. Any degree of flexion will be recorded as a positive number, e.g. 10, 20 degrees etc. In cases where the full knee extension is achieved without thigh movement, the knee is flexed and the thigh is moved to 30 degrees past the vertical position, and the knee again straightened. The angle of knee flexion at which the thigh begins to move is again recorded.

20

Abdominal Curl Conditioning Test

This commercially available abdominal test measures the muscular strength and endurance of the abdominal muscles and hip-flexors using a pre-recorded tempo.

- **Purpose:** The curl up test measures abdominal strength and endurance, which is important in back support and core stability.
- **Equipment required:** gym mat or similar, tape recorder or CD player, NCF Abdominal Curl Conditioning Test audio tape or CD version (package consists of the audio cassette or cd and booklet, The booklet describes the function and importance of the abdominal muscles and suggests useful exercises).
- **Description / procedure:** The detailed instructions on how to perform the test is included in the booklet and on the recording. Subjects are required to perform as many sit ups as possible, keeping in time to the audio recording. The test is over when the subject is not able ot perofrm the sit up in time with the bveeps, or is not able to perform the correct technique.

- **Scoring:** The total number of correctly performed sit ups that were performed in time with the beeps is recorded. Using this number and the scale below, a rating score can be derived.

Table 10. Abdominal Curl

Stage	*Total sit ups*	*Males*	*Females*
1	20	Poor	Poor
2	42	Poor	Fair
3	64	Fair	Fair
4	89	Fair	Good
5	116	Good	Good
6	146	Good	Very Good
7	180	Excellent	Excellent
8	217	Excellent	Excellent

- **Advantages:** this test is simple and quick to perform requiring minimal equipment, and large groups may be tested at once.
- **Disadvantages:** It is sometimes difficult to determine if a correct sit up is performed, and there may be dispute about the total score. The instructor should make it clear to the athlete of when they will terminate the test. As the tape may stretch over time, or the tape player may not be properly calibrated, the cd version is the preferred choice.
- **Comments:** As the audio-tapes may stretch over time, the tapes need to be calibrated. There is a one-minute interval on the tape and instructions on making adjustment to the distance between markers based on this.

21

Sit-Up / Crunch Test

This is a general description of a sit up test to measure abdominal muscle endurance. The procedures and technique can vary depending on which specific test you are performing. There is also test instructions for specific abdominal endurance tests: President's Challenge Curl Up, NCF Abdominal Conditioning Test, Home Sit Up Test, and the 2-minute tests used for the US Army, US Navy and US Marines.

- **Purpose:** The curl up test measures abdominal muscular strength and endurance of the abdominals and hip-flexors, important in back support and core stability.
- **Eequipment required:** flat, clean, cushioned surface, stopwatch, recording sheets, pen. Some variations will also require a metronome (or audio tape, cd, drums).
- **Sit-up technique:** Described here are the commonly used methods and some general guidelines. The subject lies on a cushioned, flat, clean surface with knees flexed, usually at 90 degrees. Some techniques may specify how far the feet are from the buttocks, such as about 12 inches. A partner may assist by anchoring the feet to the ground. The position of the hands and arms can affect the difficulty of the test. They should not be placed behind the head as this encourages the subject to stress the neck and pull the head forward. The hand may be placed by the side of the head, or the arms crossed over

the chest or reaching out in front. The subject raises the trunk in a smooth motion, keeping the arms in position, curling up to touch their hands or chest to the knees. The trunk is lowered back to the floor so that the shoulder blades or upper back touch the floor.

Test procedure: The maximum number of sit ups performed in a certain time period (such as one or two minutes) is recorded. Alternatively, the test may be performed at a set tempo, and the maximum number of total situps is recorded. For this method, a metronome may be set at the desired tempo, or a audio tape or cd with a recording of the pace may be used.

Scoring: The completion of one complete curl up (up and back) counts as one. The situp must be performed correctly for it to be counted. For the tempo tests, the test is continued until the subject cannot maintain the rhythm or has reached the target number for the test.

Advantages: this test is simple to perform requiring minimal equipment, and large groups may be tested at once.

Disadvantages: a curl up with the feet held increases the involvement of the hip flexor muscles, making the test less valid as a measure of abdominal strength. It is sometimes difficult to determine if a correct sit up is performed, and there may be dispute about the total number. When using the tempo method, the instructor should have clear guidelines of when they terminate the test.

Comments: Make sure that the subject does not "bounce" off the floor - only correctly performed curl ups should be counted. The partner may assist by counting aloud the number of repetitions. It is important that the correct technique is used as described for accurate comparison to the norms. If using a variation of the test, the actual technique and procedure should be recorded with the results, and appropriate norm tables consulted.

Guidelines: before conducting any fitness test, you should review each person's medicals.

22

Abdominal Strength Test - Straight Leg Lift

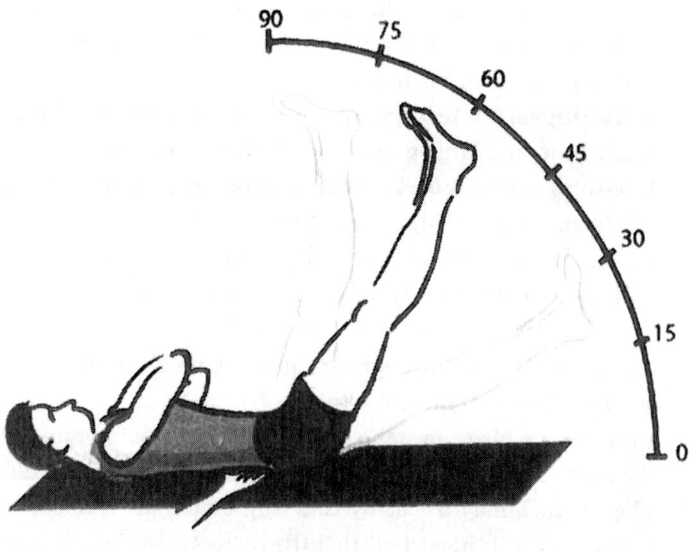

Fig. 11. Leg Lift

- **Purpose:** The purpose of this test is to estimate the degree of abdominal strength. Poor abdominal muscle strength can cause poor posture leading to lower back pain.
- **Equipment required:** flat surface, an abdominal strength test board with different degrees of angle marked (otherwise,

you can use a protractor, flexometer or goniometer to measure the leg angle)

Description / procedure: The subject lays supine on the floor next to the abdominal strength test board. The hip joint should be aligned to the intersection of the scale. The arms are held across the chest and the head rested on the floor. The testor places their finger tips underneath the subject's lower back. Both legs are raised to a 90-dregee angle (vertically) while keeping the upper body flat on the floor. The subject may bend their knees first to move to the starting position, before straightening the knee joint. The subject aims to sustain the pressure on the testor's fingers under the lower back by contracting the abdominals as the legs are lowered. The subject slowly lowers both legs until the pressure on the hand behind the back disappears. The lowest angle observed as the pressure is taken off is the measurement of their abdominal strength.

- **Scoring:** The score is the angle of the legs in degrees from the floor. Below is a guide to scoring for this test

Table 11 Straight Leg Lift

Angle	*Rating*
90	very poor, starting position
75	poor
60	below average
45	average
30	above average
15	good
0	excellent, legs horizontal

- **Advantages:** simple test with minimal equipment needed
- **Comments:** The muscles that play a major role in the effort to maintain the position of the low back and pelvis during the leg-lowering movement are the rectums abdominals and external oblique muscles.

23

Aero Test

The Aero test is variation of the popular bleep/beep/multistage fitness test for measuring aerobic fitness. For more information, the complete guide to the beep test can be found here.

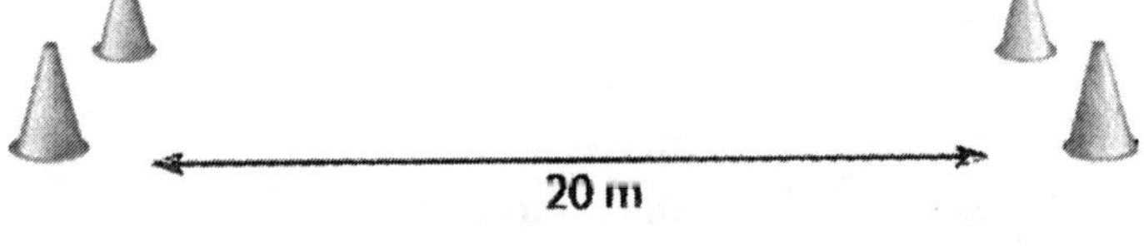

Fig. 12. Marking Cones -1

Description: Use cones to mark out two lines 20 meters apart. The subject starts on or behind one of the lines, and begins running when instructed by the cd. This subject continues running between the two lines, turning when signaled by the recorded beeps. Each bleep is 0.05 km/hr quicker than the last one, and each 20 meters that is run counts as a score of one. If the line is not reached in time the subject must run to the line turn and try to catch up with the pace within 2 more 'beeps'. The test is stopped if the subject fails to catch up with the pace within the two ends.

Scoring: The athletes score is the total number of shuttles reached before they were unable to keep up with the recording. This score can be converted to a VO2max equivalent score using the following formula.

VO2max (ml / kg / min) = 5.73 x peak speed (km / hr) - 28.15

Equipment required: Flat, non-slip surface, marking cones, 20m measuring tape, pre-recorded audio cd, cd player, recording sheets.

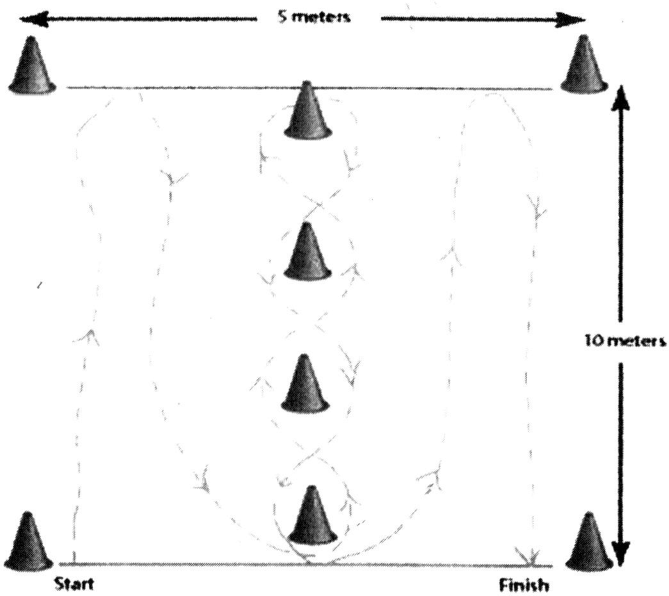

Fig. 13 : Marking Cones-2

Target population: Suitable for sports teams and school groups, but not for populations in which a maximal exercise test would be contraindicated.

Reliability: Reliability would depend on how strictly the test is run, and the practice allowed for the subjects.

Advantages: Large groups can perform this test all at once for minimal costs. Also, the test continues to maximum effort unlike many other tests of endurance capacity.

Disadvantages: Practice and motivation levels can influence the score attained, and the scoring can be subjective. As the test is usually conducted outside, the environmental conditions can be often affect the results. Norm values may be difficult to find, as it is more common to conduct the similar beep test.

Other considerations: This test is a maximal test, which requires a reasonable level of fitness. It is not recommended for recreational athletes or people with health problems, injuries or low fitness levels.

24

Shuttle Run Test

This test describes the procedures as used in the President's Challenge Fitness Awards. The variations listed give other ways to also perform this test.

Purpose: this is a test of speed and agility, important in many sports.

Equipment required: blocks, marker cones, measurement tape, stopwatch, non-slip surface.

Description / procedure: This test requires the person to run back and forth between two parallel lines as fast as possible. Set up two lines of cones 30 feet apart or use line markings, and place two blocks of wood or a similar object behind one of the lines. Starting at the line opposite the blocks, on the signal "Ready? Go!" the participant runs to the other line, picks up a block and returns to place it behind the starting line, then returns to pick up the second block, then runs with it back across the line.

Scoring: Two or more trails may be performed, and the quickest time is recorded. Results are recorded to the nearest tenth of a second.

Variations / modifications: The test procedure can be varied by changing the number of shuttles performed, the distance between turns (some use 10 meters rather than 30 feet) and by removing the need for the person pick up and return objects from the turning points.

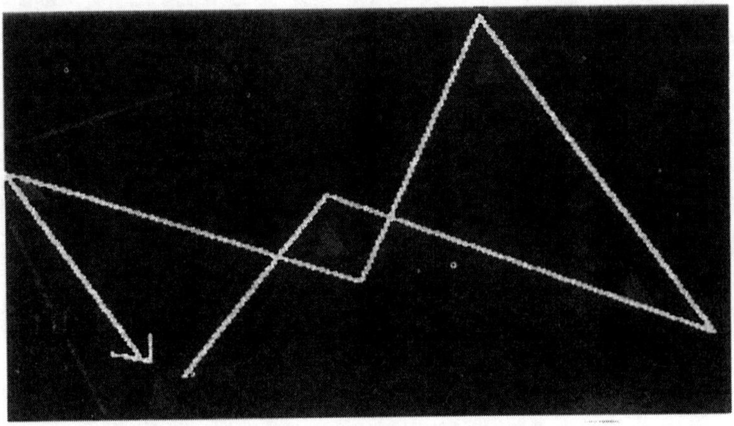

Fig. 14 : Marking Cones-3

Advantages: this test can be conducted on large groups relatively quickly with minimal equipment required.

Comments: the blocks should be placed at the line, not thrown across them. Also make sure the participants run through the finish line to maximize their score.

25

Agility Test

Eequipment required: start/stop timing gates or stopwatch, non-slip running surface, cone markers

Description / procedure: markers are set up 5 and 15 meters from a line marked on the ground. The athlete runs from the 15 meter marker towards the line (run in distance to build up speed) and through the 5 m markers, turns on the line and runs back through the 5 m markers. The time is recorded from when the athletes first runs through the 5 meter marker, and stopped when they return through these markers (that is, the time taken to cover the 5 m up and back distance - 10 m total). The best of two trails is recorded. The turning ability on each leg should be tested. The subject should be encouraged to not overstep the line by too much, as this will increase their time.

Comments: This is a test of 180 degree turning ability. This ability may not be applicable to some sports.

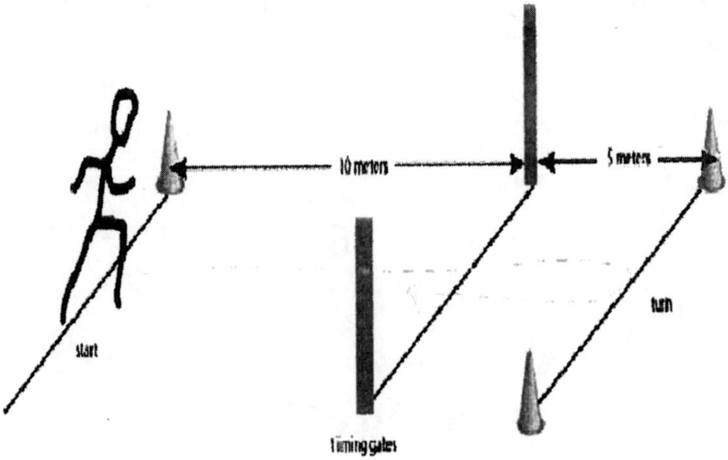

Fig. 15 : Marking Cones -4

26

Hexagon Agility Test

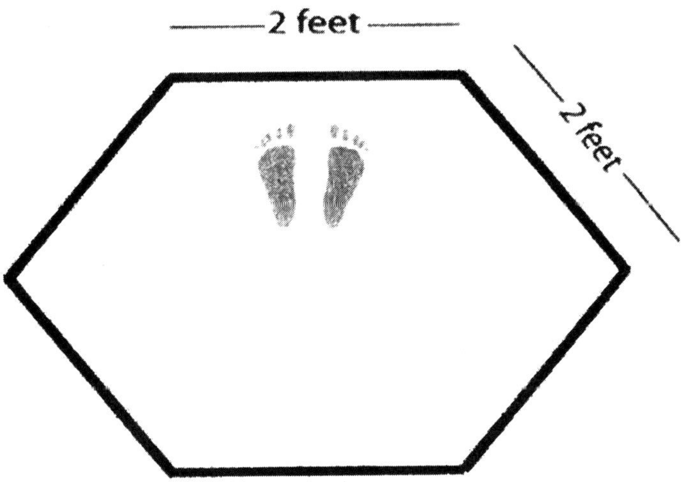

Fig. 15 : Marking Cones -4

Aim: This is a test of the ability to move with maximum speed while maintaining balance.

- **Equipment required:** tape measure, chalk or tape for marking ground, stopwatch
- **Description / Procedure:** Using athletic tape, mark a hexagon (six sided shape) on the floor. The length of each side should be 24 inches (60.5 cm), and each angle should work out to be 120 degreees. The person to be tested starts with both feet together in the middle of the hexagon facing the

front line. On the command 'go', they jump ahead across the line, then back over the same line into the middle of the hexagon. Then, continuing to face forward with feet together, jump over the next side and back into the hexagon. Continue this pattern for three full revolutions. Perform the test both clockwise and anticlockwise.

- **Scoring:** The athletes score is the time taken to complete three full revolutions. The best score from two trials is recorded. Comparison of the anticlockwise and clockwise directions will show if any imbalances exist between left and right movement skills.
- **Aadvantages:** This is a simple agility test to perform, requiring limited equipment and space.
- **Disadvantages:** Only one person can perform the test at a time.
- **Comments:** If you jump the wrong line or land on a line then the test is to be restarted

27

Back Strength Test - Isometric

- **Purpose:** this test measures back strength, which is important in for core stability and preventing lower back pain.
- **Eequipment required:** padded bench
- **Description / procedure:** Subjects must lie face down on a bench, with their upper body from the waist hanging over the end of the bench. The subjects feet must be held or strapped down, and the arms by their side or clasped behind the back. When ready, they must bring their body up to the horizontal position, and hold this for 45 seconds.
- **Scoring:** This test will be assessed as a pass or fail.
- **Advantages:** simple test to perform
- **Disadvantages:** only able to test one person at a time.
- **Variations:** the time that the horizontal position is held can be varied.

28

Balance Beam Test

- **Purpose**: To assess active balance, through the ability to maintain balance while walking along an elevated beam.
- **Equipment required:** gymnastics balance beam, stopwatch
- **Description / procedure:** The aim of this test is to walk the entire length of a standard balance beam steadily, without falling off, and within a six second time span. The participant will start at one end, step up onto the beam, walk the length to the other end. The test is repeated three times.
- **Scoring**: Participants are to be given three trials to complete the beam walk. The table below lists scores based on subjective observations of the beam walker. For more accuracy, use a team of three or more judges to observe a given individual perform. The score for each trial is the average of all the judge's scores. The overall score for the individual is the average of the three trial scores
- **Reliability:** Three judges are used to improve reliability of assessors (Inter-rater reliability), and three trials per individual are allowed to improve reliability over time (Test-retest reliability).
- **Comments:** this test can be used as a screening test for female gymnasts, as walking the beam is a basic skill for gymnastics

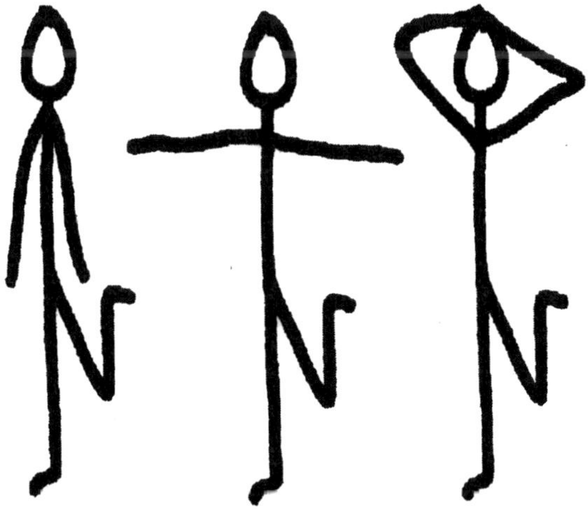

Fig. 17 : Balance Walk

29

Balance - Stork Test

- **Equipment required:** flat, non-slip surface, stopwatch, paper and pencil.
- **Description / procedure:** the person stands on one leg for as long as possible.
- **Scoring:** time length of time person can stay in balance position
- **Variations / modifications:** to increase the degree of difficulty, the test can be conducted with the person having their arms either by their sides, held out horizontally, or on their head. You could also conduct the test with their eyes closed for each of these variations too.

30

Balance Stand Test

- **Purpose**: To assess the ability to balance on the ball of the foot.
- **Equipment required:** flat, non-slip surface, stopwatch, paper and pencil.
- **Description / procedure:** Remove the shoes and place the hands on the hips, then position the non-supporting foot against

Table 12 : Balance Stand

Rating	*Score (seconds)*
Excellent	> 50
Good	40 - 50
Average	25- 39
Fair	10 - 24
Poor	< 10

the inside knee of the supporting leg. The subject is given one minute to practice the balance. The subject raises the heel to balance on the ball of the foot. The stopwatch is started as the heel is raised from the floor. The stopwatch is stopped if any of the follow occur:

- the hand(s) come off the hips
- the supporting foot swivels or moves (hops) in any direction
- the non-supporting foot loses contact with the knee.
- the heel of the supporting foot touches the floor.

- **Scoring**: The total time in seconds is recorded. The score is the best of three attempts. The table below lists general ratings for this test.

31

Balke Test Treadmill

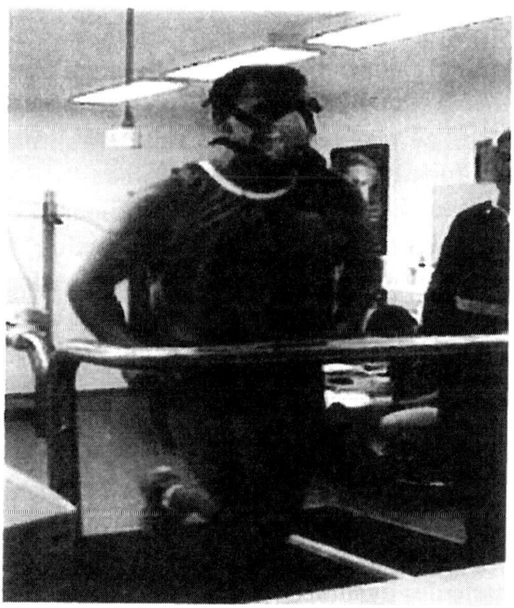

Fig. 18. Treadmill

Aim: the Balke Treadmill Test was developed as a clinical test to determine peak VO2 in cardiac patients, though it can also be used to estimate cardiovascular fitness in athletes.

Equipment required: treadmill, stopwatch, electrocardiograph (optional)

Description / procedure: (note: there is also the different Balke 15 minute run test) The athlete walks on a treadmill to exhaustion, at a constant walking speed while gradient/slope is increased every one or two minutes. The assistant starts the stopwatch at the beginning of the test and stops it when the subject is unable to continue. There are several modification or variation of the Balke test that are used, with variations in the treamill speed, time at each level and/or increase in gradient. Here are examples of test protocols that have been used.

- For men the treadmill speed is set at 3.3 mph, with the gradient starting at 0%. After 1 minute it is raised to 2%, then 1% each minute thereafter.
- For women the treadmill speed is set at 3.0 mph, with the gradient starting at 0%, and increased by 2.5% every three minutes.
- walking speed constant at 3 km/hr whilst the grade was increased by 2.5 percent every two minutes.

- **Results:** The test score is the time taken on the test, in minutes. Ideally this should be between 9-15 minutes. The test time can also be converted to an estimated VO2max score using the following formulas where the value "T" is the total time completed (expressed in minutes and fractions of a minute e.g. 9 minutes 15 seconds = 9.25 minutes) (note: only applicable if the same protocol is used as when these formula were developed):

  For men: VO2 max = 1.444 (T) + 14.99

  For women: VO2 max = 1.38 (T) + 5.22
- **Target population:** The Balke test is recommended for cardiac patients since the elevation in workload is moderate and therefore considered safe even for patients with severe left ventricular dysfunction.
- **Advantages:** You can also get measurement of maximum heart rate by recording heart rate during the test, which can be used in training programs to set intensity.
- **Disadvantages:** Relatively long time to conduct the test, and high costs involved in terms of equipment and time
- **Other comments:** Other similar exercise stress test protocols include Astrand, Naughton and Bruce. Note that there is also the field test also developed by Balke: 15 minute run test
- **Caution:** This test is a maximal test. If used recreational athletes or people with health problems, injuries or low fitness levels, please have medical assistance on hand.

32

Body Mass / Weight

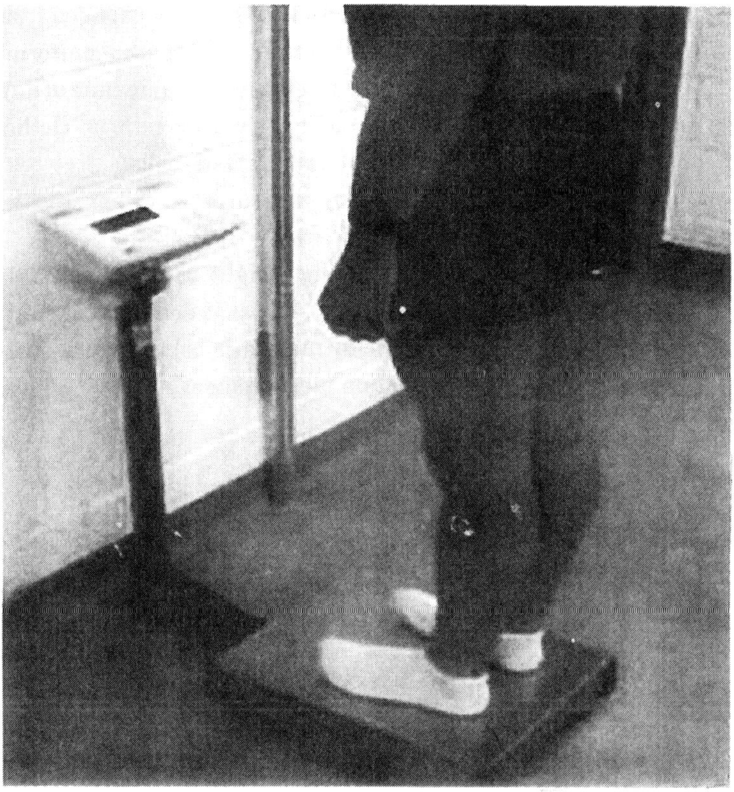

Fig. 19 : Body Weight

Purpose: measuring body mass can be valuable for monitoring body fat or muscle mass changes, or for monitoring hydration level.

Equipment required: Scales, which should be calibrated for accuracy using weights authenticated by a government department of weights and measures.

Description / procedure: the person stands with minimal movement with hands by their side. Shoes and excess clothing should be removed.

Reliability: To improve reliability, weigh routinely in the morning (12 hours since eating). Body weight can be affected by fluid in the bladder (weigh after voiding the bladder). Other factors to consider are the amount of food recently eaten, hydration level, the amount of waste recently expelled from the body, recent exercise and clothing. If you are monitoring changes in body mass, try and weigh at the same time of day, under the same conditions, and preferably with no clothes on. Always compare using the same set of scales.

Advantages: quick and easy measurement when testing large groups, with minimal costs.

Other comments: measuring weight can be used as a measure of changes in body fat, but as it does not take into account changes in lean body mass it is better to use other methods of body composition measurement.

33

Body Mass Index (BMI)

BMI stands for Body Mass Index. It is a measure of body composition. BMI is calculated by taking a person's weight and dividing by their height squared. For instance, if your height is 1.82 meters, the divisor of the calculation will be (1.82 * 1.82) = 3.3124. If your weight is 70.5 kilograms, then your BMI is 21.3 (70.5 / 3.3124) (see calculator links below).

The higher the figure the more overweight you are. Like any of these types of measures it is only an indication and other issues such as body type and shape have a bearing as well. Remember, BMI is just a guide - it does not accurately apply to elderly populations, pregnant women or very muscular athletes such as weightlifters.

Calculate your own BMI !

If you are from the US and want to enter your height in feet and inches, and weight in pounds, use this calculator.

For the rest of the world, there is a metric version for entering height in meters and weight in kilograms.

Test Details

Equipment required: scales and stadiometer as for weight and height.

Description / procedure: BMI is calculated from body mass (M) and height (H). BMI = M / (H x H), where M = body mass in kilograms and H = height in meters. The higher the score usually indicating higher levels of body fat.
Scoring: Use the table below to determine your BMI rating. You can also use an ideal height and weight graph.

Table 13 : Ideal Body Mass

	Men	*Women*
underweight	< 20	< 19
healthy range	20-25	19-24
overweight	26-30	25-30
obese	> 30	> 30

Target population: BMI is often used to determine the level of health risk associated with obesity.
Advantages: simple calculation from standard measurements
Disadvantages: BMI can be inaccurate, for example with large and muscular though lean athletes scoring high BMI levels which incorrectly rates them as obese.
Other comments: Other simple measures of body composition, such as skinfolds measures, would be preferable if available.

34

Box Drill Fitness Test

This test used to be part of the testing battery for the NFL Combine, before being replaced by the 3-Cone Drill.

Purpose: this is a test of agility, including speed, quickness, flexibility, change of direction and body control.

Equipment required: stopwatch, measuring tape, 4 marker cones, a flat non-slip surface

Description / procedure: Four marker cones are placed 10 yards apart in a square configuration (see diagram). The player starts by getting down in a three-point stance next to Cone 1. On the command 'Go', he sprints to cone 2, then shuffles sideways to cone 3. From there you back-pedal to cone 4 and finish by turning and sprinting through and finishing at cone 1. The athlete must go around the outside of each cone.

Scoring: The time to complete the test in seconds is recorded. The score is the best time of two trials.

Target population: This test used to be part part of the NFL testing combine, though it would be suitable for athletes involved in many team sports where agility is important such basketball, hockey, rugby, soccer.

Comments: The the "4 Cone" or "Box" drill has been replaced by the 3-Cone Drill in the NFL scouting combine.

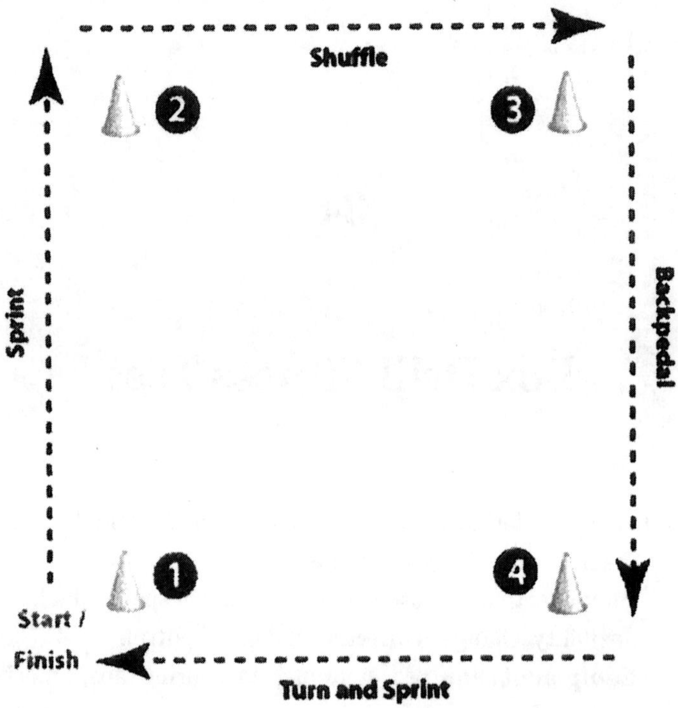

Fig. 20 : Box Drill

35

Canadian Home Fitness Test

This test was specifically developed for a fitness survey of the Canadian people in the early 1980s. It is a test of aerobic fitness which people could perform themselves at home.

- **Purpose:** for the measurement of aerobic fitness of the general population, which is important for overall health. Performing such a test has the benefit of increasing fitness awareness, and as a rough estimate of personal fitness can be used to monitor and motivate those undertaking an exercise program.
- **Description:** The test is a simple, progressive, submaximal aerobic test. Subjects step up and down a double step (40.6 cm), following the instructions and stepping rhythm as determined by recorded music (using the LP record or tape), based on their age and sex. Stepping is performed with a six pace cycle: one foot on the middle step, two on the top step, one on the middle step, and both feet on the ground. The subject starts with a warm up, stepping for 3 minutes at a rhythm appropriate to a person who is 10 years older than themselves. Pulse rate is measured for 10 seconds (between 5 & 15 seconds after stepping). If the pulse rate is within a specified safety zone, stepping is recommenced at 3 minutes 25 seconds, using a rhythm appropriate to the individual's age. After another 3 minutes of stepping, the pulse is taken

again. If the pulse ceiling still has not been reached, the subject continues for a third stage, at a stepping rate appropriate to a person who is 10 years younger than themselves.

- **Equipment required:** double 20.3 cm (8 inch) step such as may be found in most North American homes, a long-playing record or tape recording and player. If accuracy is important, the player speed should be calibrated.
- **Results:** A simple categorization of fitness is based upon the number of test stages the subject can complete and the pulse count between 5 - 15 sec following the final test stage. It is also possible to convert this score to a predicted VO2max result, using the equation by Jetté et al., 1976: VO2max = 42.5 + 16.6 (E) - 0.12 (M) - 0.12 (fh) - 0.24 (A) where VO2max is the aerobic power in ml.kg-1.min-1, E is the energy cost of the final test stage in l.min-1 (table of values needed), M is the body mass in kg, fh is the heart rate in beats.min-1 and A is the subject's age in years.
- **comments:** some practice may be required to get the required stepping frequency, and in recording the pulse rate accurately. It is important that the stepping rhythm be sustained, that the person stand upright on the top step and place both feet flat on the floor at the end of each stepping movement. The subject should also try to minimize any extraneous movements.
- **Advantages:** this test was designed to be self-administered. Other than the recording that is required, the test requires simple equipment that can be found in the home and is easy to conduct.
- **Disadvantages:** The tape or LP recording is not readily available outside of Canada.
- **Assumptions:** Like other submaximal tests of aerobic fitness, this test relies on the approximate linear relationship between exercise heart rate and oxygen intake. It is also assumed that stepping exercise is performed with a known and consistent mechanical efficiency, so that the subject's net energy expenditure can be estimated from the corresponding

stepping rate. In addition, it is assumed that there is a minimal decrease in the pulse rate in the first 15 seconds following the test, and that an 10 second pulse count can be recorded accurately.

36

Chester Step Test

- **Overview:** a sub-maximal stepping test of aerobic fitness. It is a variation of a stepping type fitness tests (see other step tests), and is commonly used in the UK.
- **Equipment:** step, heart rate monitor, portable cassette or compact disk player, and perceived exertion scale
- **Description / procedure:** The step height varies for different participants (from 0.15 to 0.30 meters) - there are standardized criteria for choosing a step height based on the subjects age and physical activity history. The initial step rate is 15 steps per minute and every 2 minutes the tempo increases by 5 steps per minute. The stepping rate is set by a recorded metronome and guided verbal instructions, which are played on a cassette tape or compact disc. When the subject reaches 80% of age estimated heart rate maximum and/or an RPE of 14 on Borg's 6–20 scale, they are told to stop the test.
- **Purchase:** The Chester Step Test (CD Rom) is available on CD, which includes metronome and music beat audio tracks plus 50 data collection sheets. The easy to use software automatically calculates your Chester Step score and stores your history data so you can monitor your progress over time. The resource manual can be viewed on screen, or alternatively can be printed off to take to your sessions.

- **Advantages:** minimal equipment is required and the test is very portable. The test is designed to be flexible in assessing people with a wide range of absolute aerobic fitness levels by having adjustable step heights.
- **Disadvantages:** for some groups, subjects may not honestly gauge their Rate of Perceived Exertion for various reasons such as saving face among peers. If the step height is not adjusted for subject age and physical activity, as is sometime done, then shorter subjects may be at a disadvantage.
- **History:** The Chester Step test was developed by Kevin Sykes while at Chester College – a College of the University of Liverpool, and was developed to assess aerobic fitness in fire brigades in Britain, Europe, USA, and Asia.

37

Hand Wall Toss Test

- **Purpose:** to measure hand-eye coordination
- **Equipment required:** tennis ball or baseball, smooth and solid wall, marking tape, stopwatch (optional)
- **Description / procedure:** A mark is placed a certain distance from the wall (e.g. 2 meters, 3 feet). The person stands behind the line and facing the wall. The ball is thrown from one hand in an underarm action against the wall, and attempted to be caught with the opposite hand. The ball is then thrown back against the wall and caught with the initial hand. The test can continue for a nominated number of attempts or for a set time period (e.g. 30 seconds). By adding the constraint of a set time period, you also add the factor of working under pressure.
- **Scoring:** The table below lists general ratings for this test, using the score of the number of successful catches in a 30 second period.
- **Variations / modifications:** There are numerous variation that can be made to the procedures of this test depending on the desired outcomes: the size, weight and shape of the object, the distance from the wall, the number of attempts or time period can all be varied. The procedure should be recorded with the results and kept consistent for future testing of the same subjects.

Table 14 : Hand Wall Toss Test Soon

Rating	*Score (in 30 seconds)*
Excellent	> 35
Good	30 - 35
Average	20- 29
Fair	15 - 19
Poor	< 15

- **Advantages:** minimal equipment and costs are involved in conducting this test, and it can be self-administered.
- **Disadvantages:** the ability to catch the ball can be affected by how hard and straight the ball is thrown to the wall. You may want to draw a target on the wall to help with throwing accuracy. The test results may be skewed if the subject 'flukes' a few catches, so repeating the test a few times may result in more accurate results.

38

Muscle Flexibility Test

Description / procedure: For each leg, stand the maximum distance you can stand flat footed away from the wall, and also be able to bend your knee to touch the wall.
Scoring: measure the maximum distance from toe to the wall. There appears to be no norms available for this test.
Equipment required: ruler or tape measure.
Disadvantages: Variations in leg length can make comparisons between individuals misleading. Unless you are testing a fairly homogenous group, it is best to use this test to monitor changes over time in the same individual.

39

Flexibility Using A Flexometer

- **Purpose:** the aim of this test is to measure the flexibility of a joint, which is important for injury prevention and execution of many sporting movements.
- **Equipment required:** Flexometer, which consists of a gravity needle and a strap which attaches to the limb. (It is also possible to use an inclinometer or clinometer, instruments designed for measuring angles of slope)
- **Description / procedure:** The flexometer is attached to the limb, and the change in angle on the flexometer is noted from one extreme position to the another
- **Reliability:** high
- **Advantages:** there is no need to identify the axis of rotation as with the goniometer.

40

Glucose Tolerance Test (GTT)

Aim: A glucose tolerance test determines how quickly glucose is cleared from the blood. The test is usually used to test for diabetes and insulin resistance.

- **Equipment required:** blood glucose analyzer, blood collection apparatus, glucose, scales.
- **Description / procedure:** The test is performed immediately following a fast of between 8-16 hours. A fasting blood glucose measurement is performed immediately prior to the test. If this level is greater than 7.0 mmol/L, the test is usually not performed as this level signifies diabetes mellitus. The patient is then given a glucose solution to drink. Adults are given 75 grams of glucose, children are given an amount dependent on their weight: 1.75 g/kg body weight (up to 75 grams maximum). The patient is instructed to rest, then another blood glucose measurement is taken after 2 hours.
- **Contraindications:** the GTT should not be done if the patient is ill, is known to have diabetes mellitus, or has symptoms suggestive of diabetes mellitus (e.g. fasting plasma glucose $\geq$7.0 mmol/L or random plasma glucose $\geq$11.1 mmol/L.

Table 15 : Glucose Tolerance Test

Rating	*Fasting*	*2 Hour*
Normal	< 5.5 mmol/L	< 7.8 mmol/L
Impaired glucose tolerance	< 5.5 mmol/L	7.8 - 11.0 mmol/L
Impaired fasting glycemia	5.5 - 6.9 mmol/L	< 7.8 mmol/L
Diabetes mellitus:	≥ 7.0 mmol/L	≥ 11.1 mmol/L

41

Flexibility Using A Goniometer

- **Purpose:** the aim of this test is to measure the flexibility of a joint, which is important for injury prevention and execution of many sporting movements.
- **Equipment required:** Goniometer.
- **Description / procedure:** To measure the range of motion at a joint, the center of the goniometer is positioned at the axis of rotation of a joint, and the arms of the goniometer are aligned with the long axis of the bones of the adjacent segments or to an external reference.
- **Scoring:** The measurement is the angle in degrees as read off the goniometer.
- **Disadvantages:** It is sometimes difficult to position and maintain the arms of the goniometer along the bones of the segments throughout the measurement, and the axis of rotation is not always clear, especially for complex joints.

42

Flexibility Test Girth - arm-flexed

- **Purpose:** This simple test measures the flexibility in the adductor muscles.
- **Equipment required:** ruler or tape measure.

Table 16 : Arm Girth

Ratings	*Score*
Excellent	5 cm
Good	10 cm
Very Good	15 cm
Fair	20 cm
Poor	25 cm

- **Description / procedure:** Sit on the floor with your knees bent, and your feet flat on the floor and legs together. Let your knees drop sideways as far as possible keeping your feet together. The soles of your feet should be together and facing each other. Hold on to your feet with both hands, and pull you ankles as close to your body as possible. Measure the distance from your heels to your groin.

- **Scoring:** Use the table below to convert the score measurement to a rating.
- **Advantages:** simple and quick test to perform. Athletes can perform the test themselves.

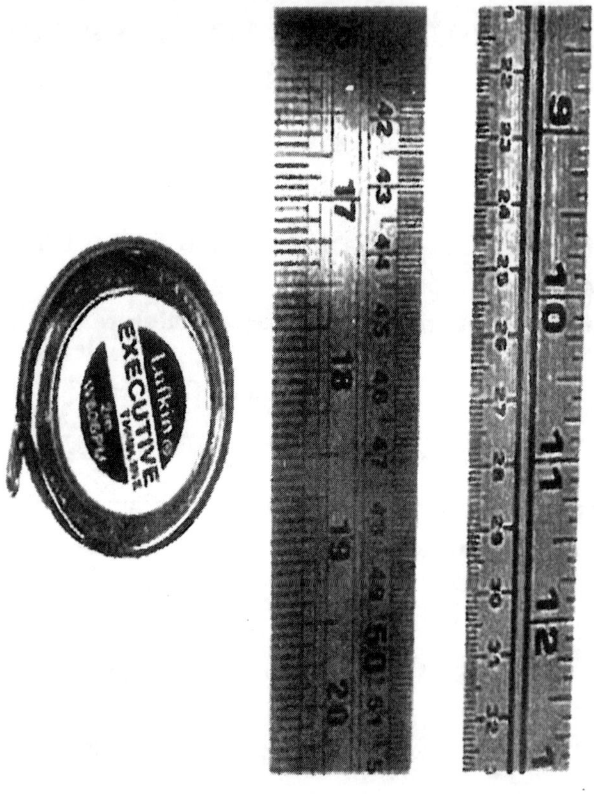

Fig. 21 : Ruler

43

Span

- **Purpose:** The size of the hand is advantageous for some sports which involve catching, gripping or tackling.
- **Equipment required:** flat surface and ruler or tape measure
- **Description / procedure:** The hand is placed palm down on a flat surface. The fingers are outstretched as far as possible. Measure the linear distance between the outside of the thumb to the outside of the little finger.
- **Advantages:** very low cost, simple and quick test
- **Other comments:** this test is used at the AFL Draft Camp

44

Step Test

- **Aim:** the purpose of this test is to determine aerobic fitness using a simple test and minimal equipment.
- **Equipment required:** step or platform 20 inches / 50.8 cm high, stopwatch, metronome or cadence tape.
- **Description / procedure:** The athlete steps up and down on the platform at a rate of 30 steps per minute (every two seconds) for 5 minutes or until exhaustion. Exhaustion is defined as when the athlete cannot maintain the stepping rate for 15 seconds. The athlete immediately sits down on completion of the test, and the total number of heart beats are counted between 1 to 1&frac12 minutes after finishing. This is the only measure required if using the *short form* of the test. If the *long form* of the test is being conducted, there is an additional heart rate measures at between 2 to 2&frac12 minutes, and between 3 to 3&frac12 minutes.
- **Scoring:** the Fitness Index score is determined by the following equations. For example, if the total test time was 300 seconds (if completed the whole 5 minutes), and the number of heart beats between 1-1&frac12 minutes was 90, between 2-2&frac12 it was 80 and between 3-3&frac12 it was 70, then the long form Fitness Index score would be: (100 x

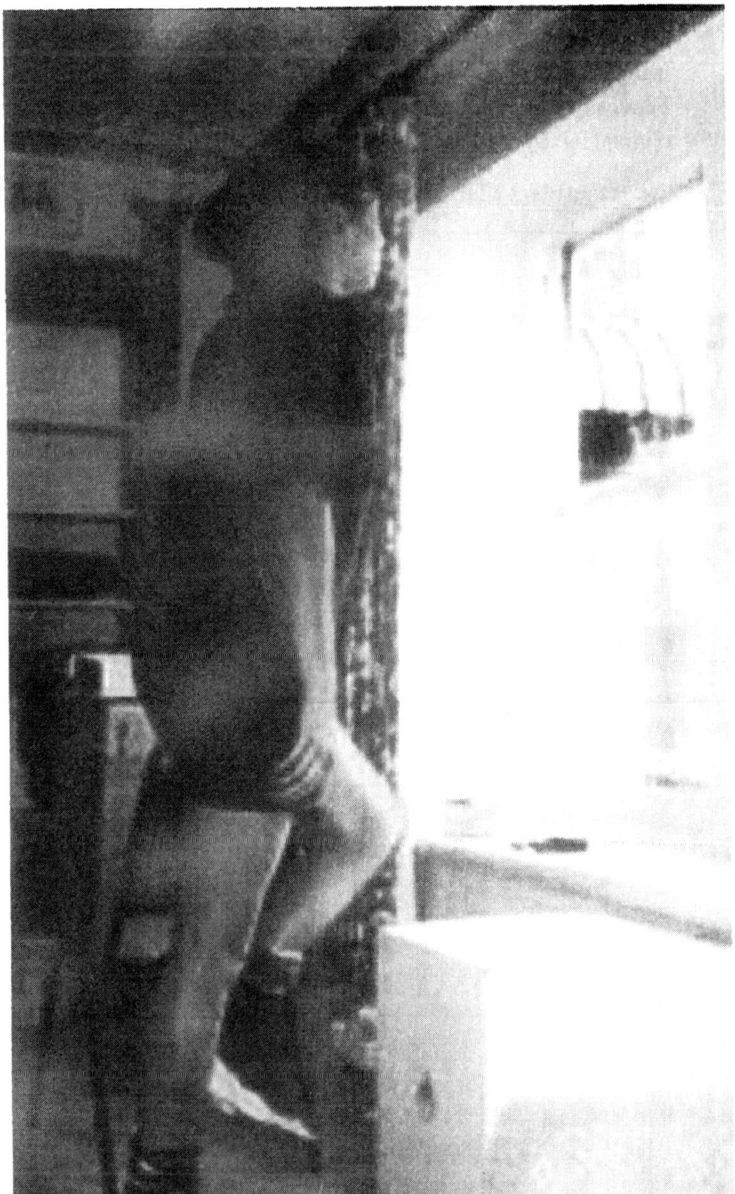

Fig. 22 : Step Test

300) / (240 x 2) = 62.5. Note: you are using the total number of heart beats in the 30 second period, not the rate (beats per minute) during that time.

- ***Fitness Index*** (short form) = (100 x test duration in seconds) divided by (5.5 x pulse count between 1 and 1&frac12 minutes).

Table 17 : Fitness Index - Short Form

Rating	*Fitness Index (Long Form)*
good	> 80
average	50 - 80
poor	< 50

- ***Fitness Index*** (long form) = (100 x test duration in seconds) divided by (2 x sum of heart beats in the recovery periods).

Table 18 : Fitness Index - Long Form

Rating	*Fitness index (long form)*
excellent	> 90
good	80 - 89
high average	65 - 79
low average	55 - 64
poor	< 55

- **Validity:** correlation to VO_{2max} approximately 0.6 to 0.8
- **Advantages:** This test requires minimal equipment and costs, and can be self-administered.
- **Disadvantages:** Biomechanical characteristics vary between individuals. For example, considering that the step height is standard, taller people are at an advantage as it will take less energy to step up onto the step. Body weight has also been

shown to be a factor. Testing large groups with this test will be time consuming.

- **Comments:** The Harvard Step Test was developed by Brouha et al. (1943) in the Harvard Fatique Laboratories during WWII. Some sources suggest a 40 cm high bench, which is not the standard and original bench height. Since the original description of this test, there have been variations in the test procedure such as reducing the bench height for female subjects in some research studies. Also be aware that I have noticed that some websites incorrectly list the formula for the long form without doubling the demonimator.

45

Height - Sitting

- **Description / procedure:** Sitting height gives a measure of the length of the trunk. It is a measurement of the distance from the highest point on the head to the base sitting surface. The subject sits with both feet on the floor, the lower back and shoulders against the wall, looking straight ahead. Distance can be measured from the floor, and the height of the box measured and subtracted from the total distance.
- **Equipment required:** stadiometer or ruler placed against a wall, box or chair.
- **Reliability:** Height measurement can vary throughout the day, being higher in the morning, so should be measured at a consistent time of day.
- **Advantages:** low costs, quick test.
- **Other comments:** Upper body length or proportionally long legs is an important attribute for many sports.

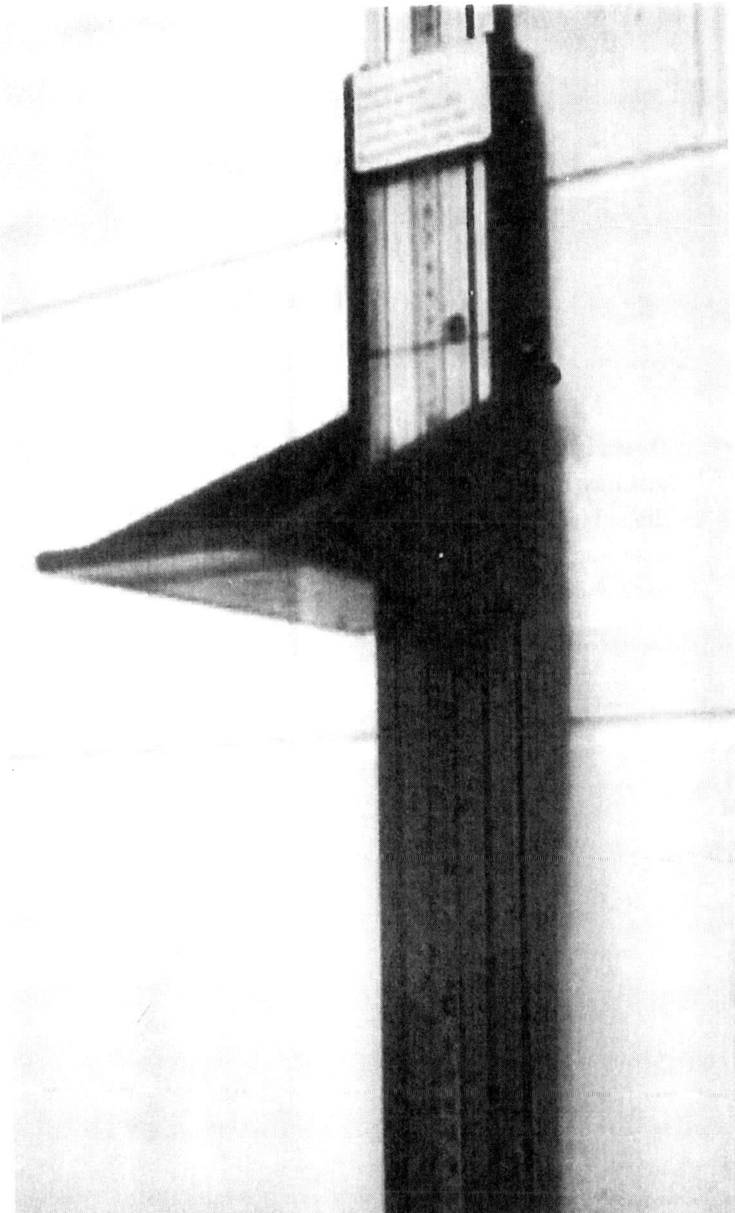

Fig. 23 : Stadiometer

46

Height - Standing

Description / procedure: measurement the maximum distance from the floor to the highest point on the head, when the subject is facing directly ahead. Shoes should be off, feet together, and arms by the sides. Heels, buttocks and upper back should also be in contact with the wall.

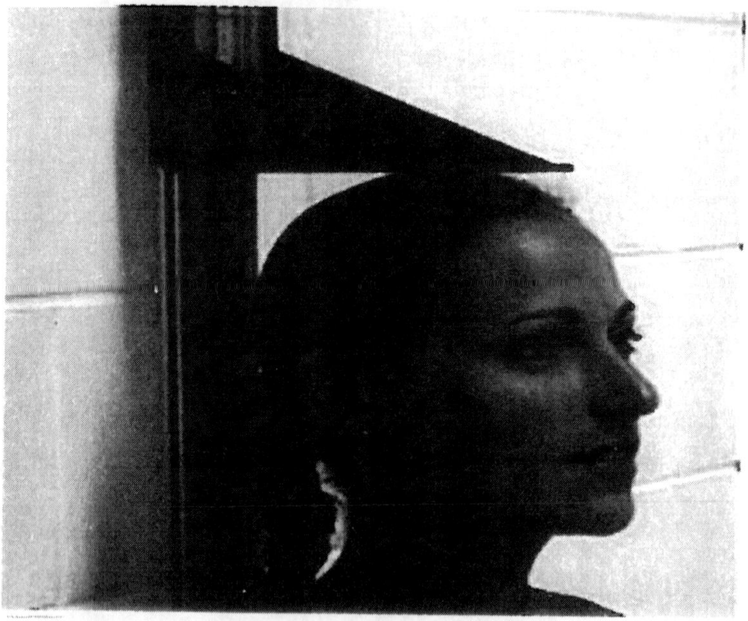

Fig. 24 : Height Standing

- **Equipment required:** stadiometer or steel ruler placed against a wall
- **Reliability:** Height measurement can vary throughout the day, being higher in the morning, so it should be measured at the same time of day each time.
- **Advantages:** low costs, quick test
- **Other comments:** height or lack of height is an important attribute for many sports.

47

Weighing

- **Purpose:** the aim of underwater weighing is to measure the density of the body, and from that figure calculate percentage body fat.
- **Equipment required:** Hydrostatic stainless steel weighing tank, including underwater mounted chair and scale, weighted belt and nose clip. A more simple set up may include a chair and scale suspended from a diving board over a pool or hot tub.
- **Description / procedure:** The dry weight of the subject is first determined. The subject, in minimal clothing, then sits on a specialized seat, expels all the air from their lungs, and is lowered into the tank until all body parts are emerged. The person must remain motionless underwater while the underwater weight is recorded. This procedure is repeated several times to get a dependable underwater weight measure.
- **Scoring:** Body density = Wa / (((Wa - Ww) / Dw) - (RV + 100cc)), where Wa = body weight in air (kg), Ww = body weight in water (kg), Dw = density of water, RV = residual lung volume, and 100cc is the correction for air trapped in the gastrointestinal tract. The body density (D) can be converted to percent bodyfat (%BF) using the Siri equation.

- **Advantages:** Underwater weighing is the most widely used test of body density and in the past was the criterion measure for other indirect measures.
- **Disadvantages:** The equipment required to do underwater weighing is expensive. The tanks are mostly located at university or other research institutions, and there is generally not easy access for the general population.
- **Validity:** This method may underestimate body fat percentage of athletes as they tend to have denser bones and muscles than non-athletes, and may overestimate body fat percentage of elderly patients suffering from osteoporosis.
- **Other comments:** Residual lung volume (RV) is required for the calculation. For more accuracy it should be physically measured, though there are calculations for RV estimation. One estimation of residual volume is one third of forced vital capacity (FVC). See lung function tests. This method is also known as Hydrodensitometry or underwater weighing.

48

Strength Tests

- **Equipment required:** Isokinetic testing equipment (e.g. Biodex, Cybex)
- **Description / procedure:** The subject is positioned so that the body movement to be measured is isolated. The equipment is then set at different speeds and the force applied can be measured throughout the range of movement.
- **Results**: The results are often reported at different speeds so that a speed/strength/power relationship can be seen. Comparison of the relative strengths of the different sides of the body, or agonists versus antagonists (e.g. quads & hamstrings) can show specific muscular limitations.
- **Advantages**: nearly any joint action can be tested by the adjustment of the equipment.
- **Disadvantages:** The equipment required is bulky and expensive.
- **Comments**: these tests are often performed at universities as part of research projects, or as part of injury rehabilitation services.

49

J.A.M. Intermittent Test

The J.A.M. Intermittent Test is a test developed to measure the intermittent fitness ability of team sport athletes. There is another somewhat similar test, the Yo-Yo Intermittent test.

- **Purpose:** The test evaluates an individual's ability to repeatedly perform intervals over a prolonged period of time.
- **Equipment required:** Flat, non-slip surface, marking cones, measuring tape, JAM test cd, cd player, recording sheets.
- **Description:** A full description of the test procedures is available with the cd and associated booklet. Cones need to be set out in a triangular circuit, the sides of different lengths. The test involves a series of walk–jog–run shuttles. The participants loop around the triangle, either running, walking or jogging in that order. Approximately every 2 minutes the run is replaced with a maximal 12 meter sprint bout. The test continues around a triangular circuit, with participants keeping in time with a series of audio signals. The time between beeps gets progressively shorter, and the test continues until the participants cannot longer keep up with the test

- **Scoring:** Your score is the time completed on the test. A minimum of 12 minutes on this test is required to get on to the National RFU TJ Panel.
- **Target population:** This test was specifically developed for assessing the fitness of Rugby Football Union Referees, but would be suitable for other team sports such as football, rugby, AFL, field hockey, team handball and basketball. The test is suitable for athletes of all levels.
- **Reliability:** The reliability would depend on how strictly the test is run, and the previous practice allowed for the subjects.
- **Advantages:** The test is easy to conduct. Large groups can perform this test all at once for minimal costs (once the kit has been bought).
- **Disadvantages:** Practice and motivation levels can influence the score attained, and the scoring of when a person cannot keep in time with the test can be subjective. As the test is usually conducted outside, the environmental conditions can also affect the results.
- **Other considerations:** This test is a maximal test, which requires a reasonable level of fitness. It is not recommended for recreational athletes or people with health problems, injuries or low fitness levels.

50

Leg Strength Test - Isometric

Purpose: this test measures back and leg strength

Equipment required: strength dynamometer, usually composed of a cable tensiometer

Description / procedure: Make sure the dial is reset to zero before you start. Stand upright on the base of the dynamometer with your feet shoulder width apart. Let your arms hang straight down to hold the center of the bar with both hands, and with the palms facing toward the body. Adjust the chain so that the knees are bent at approximately 110 degrees. In this position your back should be bent slightly forward at the hips, your head should be held upright, and you should look straight ahead. Then without bending your back, pull as hard as possible on the chain and try to straighten your legs, keeping your arms straight. Pull against the weight steadily (no jerky movements), keeping the feet flat on the base of the dynamometer. Maximum performance will result when your legs are almost straight at the end of the lift. If not, adjust the chain length and starting position.

Scoring: read the result from the dynamometer

Advantages: this is a simple test to perform

- **Disadvantages:** it is only possible to test one person at a time. The equipment is not readily available
- **Variations:** different muscle groups can be tested by adjusting the length of the chain, and the degree of leg bend.

51

Resonance Imaging (Mri)

- **Aim:** MRI is a noninvasive, painless medical test, that is used to diagnose and treat medical conditions. In terms of body composition, the high-quality images can be processed to differentiate and measure the amounts of fat and lean body tissue and teir distribution.
- **Equipment required:** MRI
- **Method:** MRI is an X-ray based method, in which a magnetic field 'excites' water and fat molecules in the body, producing a measurable signal.
- **Description / procedure:** A person lies within the magnet as a computer scans the body, which can take about 30 minutes. High-quality images show the amount of fat and where it is distributed.
- **Advantages:** this is a noninvasive method for body composition analysis
- **Disadvantages:** The use of MRI is limited due to the high cost of equipment and analysis.
- **Other comments:** the x-rays used for this technique are very safe as the equipment uses no ionizing radiation.

52

Oxygen Consumption Test (VO2max)

The VO2max test is the criterion measure of aerobic power in athletes. Described here is the method to measure VO2max directly. Many other aerobic fitness tests estimate VO2max score from their results. See the other tests of Aerobic Endurance.

- **Equipment required:** Oxygen and carbon dioxide analyzers, ergometer on which workload may be modified, stopwatch. Expired air may be collected and volume measured via Douglas bags or a Tissot tank, or measured by a pnuemotach or turbine ventilometer.
- **Description / procedure:** Exercise is performed on an appropriate ergometer (treadmill, cycle, swim bench). The exercise workloads are selected to gradually progress in increments from moderate to maximal intensity. Oxygen uptake is calculated from measures oxygen and carbon dioxide in the expired air and minute ventilation, and the maximal level is determined at or near test completion.
- **Scoring:** Results are presented as either l/min (liters per minute) or ml/kg/min (mls of oxygen per kilogram of body weight per minute). The athlete is considered to have reached

their VO_{2max} if several of the following occurred: a plateau or 'peaking over' in oxygen uptake, maximal heart rate was reached, attainment of a respiratory exchange ratio of 1.15 or greater, and volitional exhaustion. Adult norm values are available here.

- **Target population:** Any sport in which aerobic endurance is a component, such as distance runners.
- **Advantages:** This test actually measures body oxygen consumption, which other tests try to estimate. You can also get measurement of maximum heart rate by recording heart rate during the test.
- **Disadvantages:** Relatively large time and costs required
- **Other comments:** There is often variability between the performance of different analysis systems. Stringent calibration is necessary for both the expired gas and ventilation measurement systems.
- **Caution:** This test is a maximal test, which requires a reasonable level of fitness. It is not recommended for recreational athletes or people with health problems, injuries or low fitness levels.

53

Medicine Ball Throw - Side

- **Aim:** This test measures upper and lower body stɪength and explosive power, particularly with a twisting actiɑn.
- **Equipment required:** 2-5 kg medicine ball depenling on the age and ability of the group being tested, tape meɑsure
- **Description / procedure:** The subject stands at ɪ line with the feet slightly apart, and facing the direction tc which the ball is to be thrown. Start with the ball held witl the hands just under the ball, the arms extended in front f the body. The ball is then swung back behind the body, twisting the hips and torso, then swung back vigorously to thnw the ball out as far as possible. Encourgae the subejct to ue the legs, back and arms to assist to maximizing the distance thrown, The subject is also permitted to fall forward ovr the line after the ball is released. The action is repeated on each side of the body, and three attempts are allowed each ide.
- **Scoring:** The distance from the starting positioɪ to where the ball lands is recorded. The measurement is recorded to the nearest 0.5 foot or 10 cm. The best result of thee throws is used.
- **Target population:** sports in which upper body srength is important, such as rowing, tennis, javelin throwin

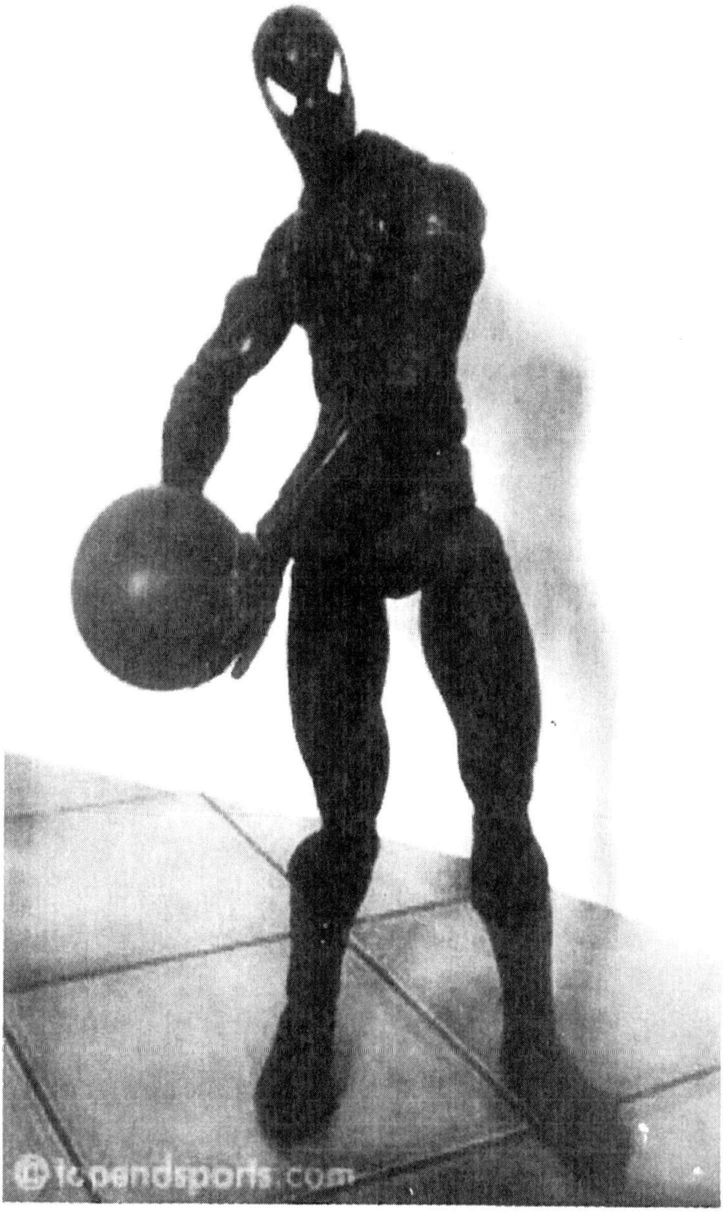

Fig. 25 : Medicine Ball Throw - Side

- **Advantages:** this test is easy and quick to perform for an individual.
- **Disadvantages:** several people are needed to conduct this test smoothly: one to mark results, another to check technique and another to collect and return the balls. If testing a large group of subjects, it can be time consuming to put all of them through this test.
- **Ccomments:** The angle the ball is thrown is important. You may want to explain to the subject about the optimal angle for maximal distance, and to allow some practice attempts. You may aid in the ease of measurement for this test by extending a tape measure out along the expected path in front of the subject. When recording the distance, you can either move the tape to where the ball landed, or less accurately align where the ball landed to the approximate distance on the tape.
- **Variations:** The weight of the medicine ball will obviously affect results, and should be selected to best test the age group or abilities of your subjects.

54

Medicine Ball Throw (Forwards)

- **Aim:** This test measures upper body strength and explosive power.
- **Equipment required:** 2-5 kg medicine ball depending on the age group being tested, tape measure
- **Description / procedure:** The subject stands at a line with the feet side by side and slightly apart, and facing the direction to which the ball is to be thrown. The ball is held with the hands on the side and slightly behind the center. The throwing action is similar to that used for a soccer/football sideline throw-in. The ball is brought back behind the head, then thrown vigorously forward as far as possible. The subject is permitted to step forward over the line after the ball is released, and is in fact encouraged to do so in maximizing the distance of the throw. Three attempts are allowed.
- **Scoring:** The distance from the starting position to where the ball lands is recorded. The measurement is recorded to the nearest 0.5 foot or 10 cm. The best result of three throws is used.
- **Target population:** sports in which upper body strength is important, such as rowing, tennis, javelin throwing

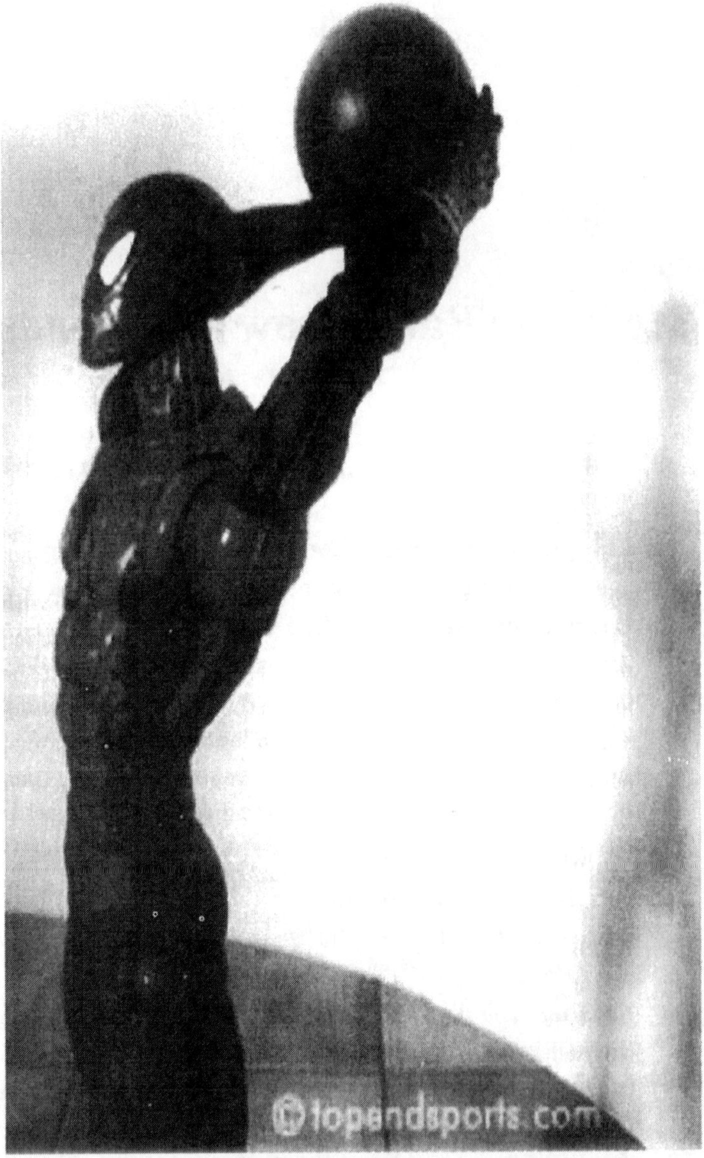

Fig. 26 : Medicine Ball Throw - Forwards

- **Advantages:** this test is easy and quick to perform for an individual.
- **Disadvantages:** several people are needed to conduct this test smoothly: one to mark results, another to check technique and another to collect and return the balls. If testing a large group of subjects, it can be time consuming to put all of them through this test.
- **Comments:** The angle that the ball is thrown is important. You may want to explain to the subject about the optimal angle for maximal distance, and to allow some practice attempts. You may aid in the ease of measurement for this test by extending a tape measure out along the expected path in front of the subject. When recording the distance, you can either move the tape to where the ball landed, or less accurately align where the ball landed to the approximate distance on the tape.
- **Variations:** Some variations of this test also allow the subject to stand at the line with one foot in front of the other. See also other medicine ball throw tests. The weight of the medicine ball will obviously affect results, and should be selected to best test the age group or abilities of your subjects.

55

Medicine Ball Throw

- **Aim:** This test measures upper and lower body strength and explosive power.
- **Equipment required:** 2 to 5 kg medicine ball (depending on the age group being tested), tape measure
- **Description / procedure:** The subject stands at a line with the feet slightly apart, and facing the direction to which the ball is to be thrown. The ball is held in both hands between the legs, with the arms extended forward and downward. The hands are placed behind and under the ball. Using the legs, back and arms to assist, the ball then thrown vigorously forward as far as possible. The subject is permitted to fall forward over the line after the ball is released, and is in fact encouraged to do so in maximizing the distance of the throw. Three attempts are allowed.
- **Scoring:** The distance from the starting position to where the ball lands is recorded. The measurement is recorded to the nearest 0.5 foot or 10 cm. The best result of three throws is used.
- **Target population:** sports in which upper body strength is important, such as rowing, tennis, javelin throwing

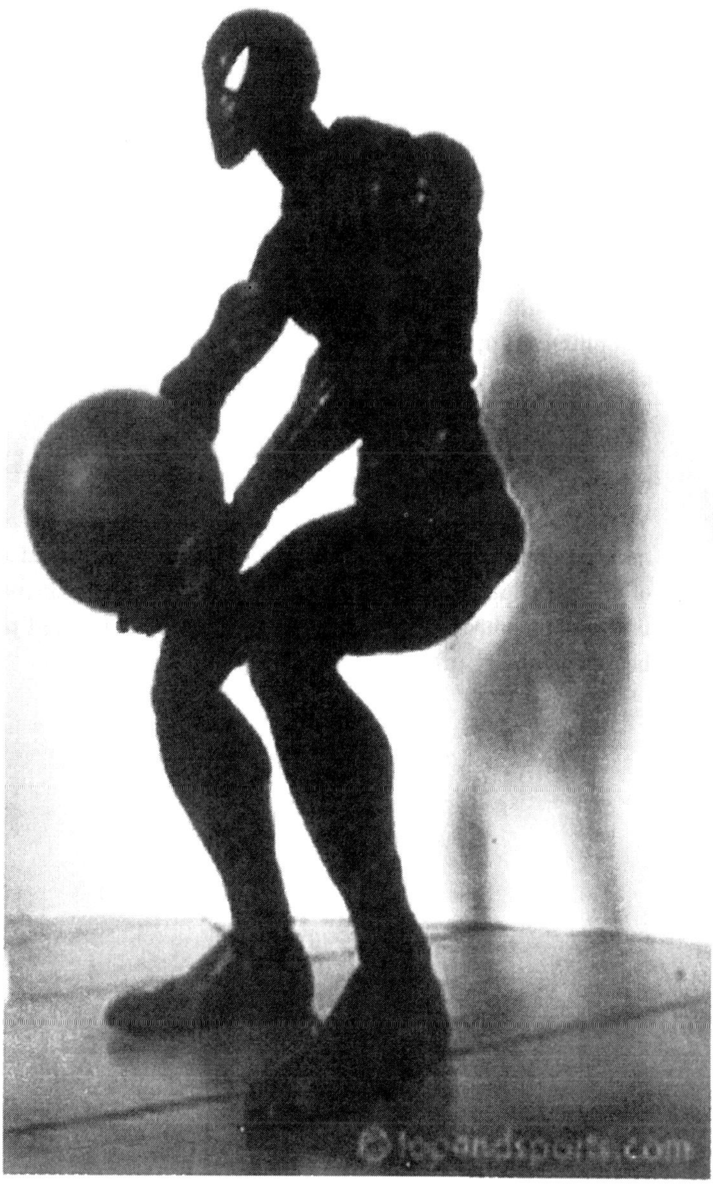

Fig. 27 : Medicine Ball Throw - Backwards

- **Advantages:** this test is easy and quick to perform for an individual.
- **Disadvantages:** several people are needed to conduct this test smoothly: one to mark results, another to check technique and another to collect and return the balls. If testing a large group of subjects, it can be time consuming to put all of them through this test.
- **Comments:** The angle the ball is thrown is important. You may want to explain to the subject about the optimal angle for maximal distance, and to allow some practice attempts. You may aid in the ease of measurement for this test by extending a tape measure out along the expected path in front of the subject. When recording the distance, you can either move the tape to where the ball landed, or less accurately align where the ball landed to the approximate distance on the tape.
- **Variations:** A similar technique can be used to throw the medicine ball toss over the head behind the subject. See also other medicine ball throw tests. The weight of the medicine ball will obviously affect results, and should be selected to best test the age group or abilities of your subjects.

56

Hurdle Jump Test

- **Purpose:** The Multistage Hurdle Test is a test of agility and lower body strength endurance, by counting the number of jumps over a hurdle in two 20 second periods and calculates a fatigue index.
- **Equipment required:** a stopwatch, SPARQ Soft Endurance Hurdle (12" high) or equivalent, 2 x timing mats (such as the JustJump) (optional).
- **Description / procedure:** Place the timing mats on either side of the hurdle. If no timing mats are available, you can manually count the number of jumps. The athlete stands comfortably on one side with both feet flat on the ground, perpendicular to the hurdle. The timing starts from the first movement. The athlete jumps off both feet and lands on both feet on the other side of the hurdle, then back again. The test continues for 20 seconds, with the total number of jumps counted. After a 20 second rest interval, the test is repeated.
- **Scoring:** The total number of completed jumps in the time period (40 seconds) is recorded, and also recovery (fatigue) index is calculated as the number of 2nd-stage jumps as a percentage of 1st stage jumps.

57

Near Infrared Interactance

- **Equipment required:** Near Infrared Interactance is measured using a computerized spectrophotometer, which has a single, rapid scanning monochromator and fiber optic probe.
- **Description / procedure:** This method uses the principles of light absorption and reflection to measure body fat. The measurement is taken on the person's dominant arm. A monochromator, or light "wand", sends a low-energy beam of near-infrared light into the biceps and penetrates the underlying tissue to a depth of one centimeter. The energy is either reflected, absorbed, or transmitted, depending on the scattering and absorption properties of the biceps. A detector within the wand measures the intensity of the re-emitted light. Shifts in the wavelength of the reflected beam and a prediction equation are used to compute the percent body fat.
- **Advantages:** The measurement is safe and the equipment is portable and lightweight. It requires little training to use.
- **Disadvantages:** This technique still lacks validation in humans, and may not accurately predict body fat across a broad range of fat levels. It assumes fat is the arm is proportional to total body fat, which may not be true.

- **Other comments:** This method is based on what was developed by the United States Department of Agriculture to measure the body composition of livestock and the fat content of various grains.
- **Products:** Futrex: uses Near-Infrared light to directly measure percent body fat.

58

Phosphate Recovery Test

Purpose: this is a test of anaerobic capacity, the ability to recover between sprints and produce the same level of power repeatedly.

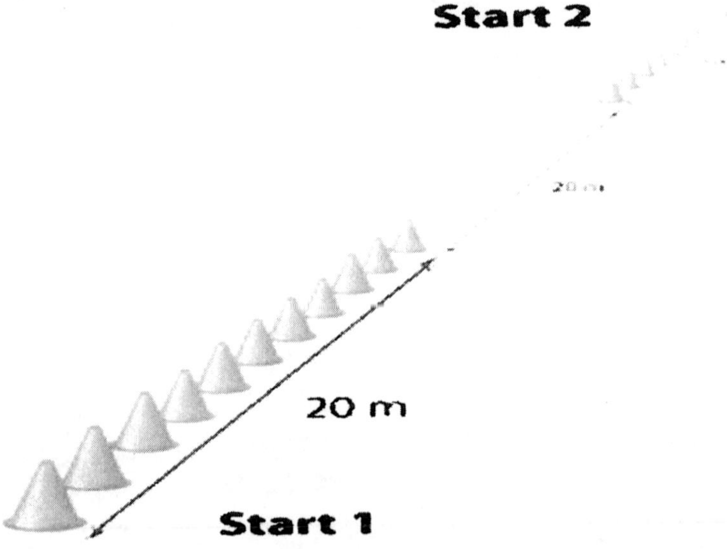

Fig. 28 : Marking Cones - 6

- **Equipment required:** Stopwatch, measuring tape, marker cones, at least 60 meter track.
- **Description / procedure:** This test involves seven all out sprints, each lasting seven seconds, with 23 seconds recovery. Marker cones are placed two meters apart for the first 20 meters. At forty meters from the first cone, cones would again be placed two meters apart to 60 meters (see diagram). The subjects set themselves at the first cone (Start 1). On the command "go", each subject would sprints 'all out' for seven seconds. At seven seconds, "time" is called and an observer would note at what cone the subject had past. The subject then has a 23 second passive recovery period before the next sprint. For the second sprint subjects would set themselves at the last cone (Start 2), facing back along the cones. At 30 seconds after the start of their first sprint, they would sprint again for seven seconds in the direction they had come. Again "time " is called at 7 seconds, and the distance run recorded. This is repeated for a total of seven sprints.
- **Scoring:** The *drop off distance* is calculated by subtracting the distance covered in the last sprint by the distance covered in the first sprint. It is expected that the last sprint would cover less distance than the other sprints due to fatigue.
- **Target population:** suitable for athletes involved in many multi-sprint sports such basketball, hockey, rugby, soccer.

59

Power Ball Chest Launch

The test involves throwing a Power Ball for maximum distance. The Kneeling Chest Launch is one of the tests of the SPARQ rating system for ice hockey and football (Gridiron), and their protocol is listed here. It is used as an alternative to the bench press in the Youth Protocol for football.

- **Aim:** This test measures upper body strength and power.
- **Equipment required:** 2 or 3 kg power ball, tape measure, foam pad for kneeling, clear open area for testing.
- **Weights:** males use 3 kg, females 2 kg, and all youth the 2 kg power ball.
- **Description / procedure:** The athlete starts by kneeling with the back erect, facing the direction they are going to throw. The thighs should be parallel and the knees at the start line. Starting with the ball grasped with both hands at the sides, and held out in front of the body. The ball is brought to the chest, then in one motion the ball is pushed forward and up (optimally at about 45 degrees). Several practices may be required to get the best trajectory for maximum distance. You must not throw favoring one arm or rotate about the spine. The athlete is permitted to fall forward over the line after the ball is released. The knees are not to leave the ground. Three attempts are allowed.

- **Scoring:** The measurement is recorded in feet and inches to the nearest inch, measuring from the outer edge of the launch line to the central point where the Power Ball first lands. The best result of three throws is recorded.
- **Target population:** football, and other sports in which upper body body power is important.
- **Advantages:** this test is easy and quick to perform for an individual, with the equipment required relatively cheap.
- **Disadvantages:** several people are needed to conduct this test smoothly: one to mark results, another to check technique and another to collect and return the balls. If testing a large group of subjects, it can be time consuming to put all of them through this test.
- **Comments:** The angle the ball is thrown is important. You may want to explain to the subject about the optimal angle for maximal distance, and to allow some practice attempts.

60

Power Ball Throw

The Rotational Power Ball Throw is one of the tests of the SPARQ rating system for baseball and hockey, and the SPARQ protocol is listed here.

- **Aim:** This test measures core strength and total body power. For baseball players, it simulates the rotational core movement common to the sport.
- **Equipment required:** 2 or 3 kg power ball (baseball uses a 3kg ball, fastpitch uses a 2 kg ball), tape measure, clear open area for testing
- **Description / procedure:** The test involves throwing a Power Ball across the chest for maximum distance. The athlete starts by standing perpendicular to the start line (such as in a pitching or hitting stance). The ball is held in both hands with the back hand on the back of the ball and your front hand under the ball. The ball is drawn back, with only a slight bend at the elbows allowed, keeping the ball between the waist and chest. Then in one motion the ball is flung up and forward (optimally at a 45 degree angle). Several practices may be required to get the best trajectory for maximum distance. The athlete is permitted to fall forward over the line after the ball is released,

and is in fact encouraged to do so in maximizing the distance of the throw. Three attempts are allowed.

- **Scoring:** The distance from the starting line to where the ball first lands is recorded. The measurement is recorded to the nearest foot. The best result of three throws is recorded.
- **Target population:** baseball, fastpitch, and other sports in which upper body strength is important, such as rowing, tennis, javelin throwing.
- **Advantages:** this test is easy and quick to perform for an individual, with the equipment required relatively cheap.
- **Disadvantages:** several people are needed to conduct this test smoothly: one to mark results, another to check technique and another to collect and return the balls. If testing a large group of subjects, it can be time consuming to put all of them through this test.
- **Comments:** The angle the ball is thrown is important. You may want to explain to the subject about the optimal angle for maximal distance, and to allow some practice attempts.

61

Ball Throw (Backwards)

The test involves throwing a Power Ball for maximum distance. The Overhead Power Ball Throw is one of the tests of the SPARQ rating system for basketball and soccer, and their protocol is listed here.

- **Aim:** This test measures core strength and total body power.
- **Equipment required:** 2 or 3 kg power ball (boys use a 3 kg, girls and youth use 2 kg), tape measure, clear open area for testing.
- **Description / procedure:** The athlete starts by standing facing away from the direction they are going to throw, with their heels at the start line. The starting position is with the ball in both hands, held above the head, with arms extended. Keeping the arms extended, swing the ball down between your legs while flexing the knees. Then in one motion the ball is flung up and back over the head (optimally at about 45 degrees). Several practices may be required to get the best trajectory for maximum distance. The athlete is permitted to fall backward over the line after the ball is released. Three attempts are allowed.

- **Scoring:** The distance from the starting line to where the ball first lands is recorded. The measurement is recorded to the nearest foot. The best result of three throws is recorded.
- **Target population:** basketball, and other sports in which total body power is important.
- **Advantages:** this test is easy and quick to perform for an individual, with the equipment required relatively cheap.
- **Disadvantages:** several people are needed to conduct this test smoothly: one to mark results, another to check technique and another to collect and return the balls. If testing a large group of subjects, it can be time consuming to put all of them through this test.
- **Comments:** The angle the ball is thrown is important. You may want to explain to the subject about the optimal angle for maximal distance, and to allow some practice attempts.

62

Chin Up Test

Objective

The objective of the Chins Test is to monitor the development of the athlete's arm and shoulder muscular endurance.

Required Resources

To undertake this test you will require :

Chinning bar

Assistant

How to conduct the test

The Chins Test is conducted as follows:

Hang from the bar with your palms facing your body

Pull up until your chin is level with the bar

Lower so as to straighten your arms

Repeat as many chins as possible

Record the number of chins

Analysis

Analysis of the result is by comparing it with the results of previous tests. It is expected that, with appropriate training between each test, the analysis would indicate an improvement.

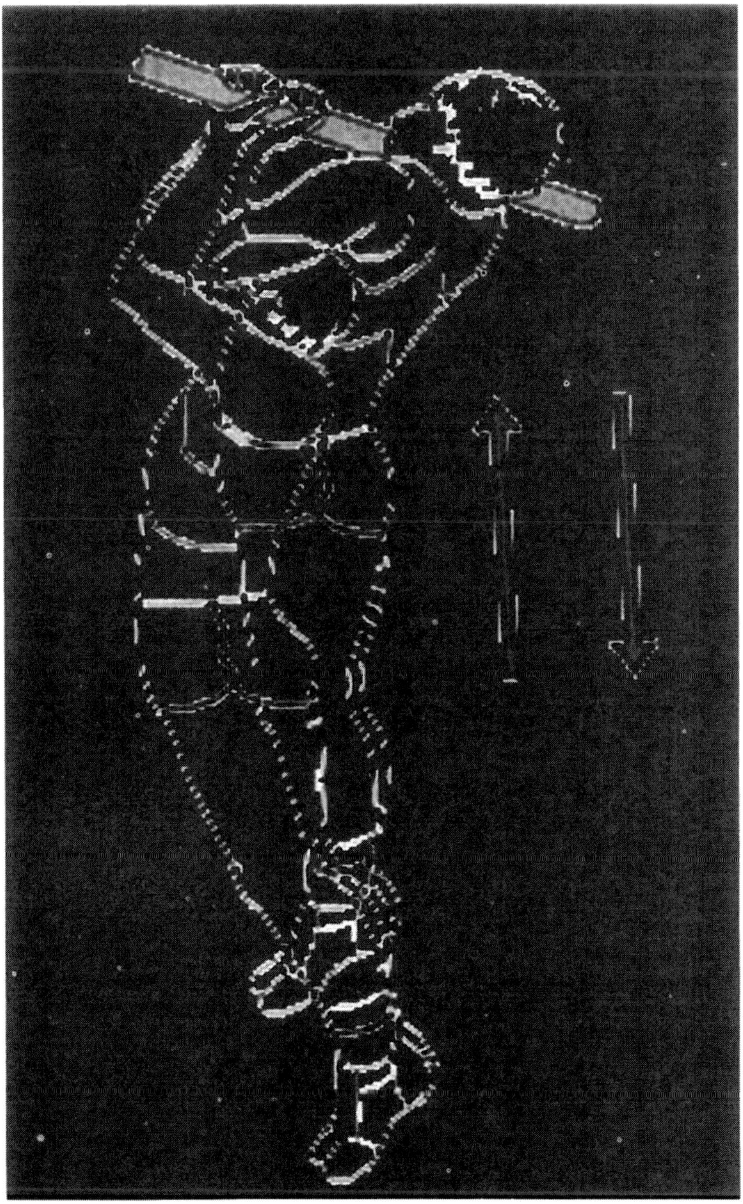

Fig. 29 : Chin Up

Normative data for the Chins test

The following are national norms for ages 16 to 19.

Table 19 : Chin Up Norms

Gender	*Excellent*	*Above average*	*Average*	*Below average*	*Poor*
Male	>13	9 - 13	6 - 8	3 - 5	<3
Female	>6	5 - 6	3 - 4	1 - 2	0

63

Pull Up Test

This test forms part of the US Marine Physical Fitness Test (PFT), performed by US Marine personnel every six months. The pull up test is only performed by the male Marines. Females perform the flexed arm hang test.

- **Purpose:** This test measures upper body strength and endurance.
- **Equipment required:** Horizontal overhead bar, at an adequate height so that the participants can hang from with arms fully extended and feet not touching the floor.
- **Description / procedure:** The pull-ups are performed starting from a dead hang (arms fully extended and locked), body motionless, feet off the floor. The grip can be either with both palms facing forward or to the rear, though with both facing in the same direction. From this starting position, a pull-up is performed without excessive body motion, and the body is lifted until the chin has cleared the top of the bar. The body is then lowered until his arms are fully extended or locked out. One complete pull-up is counted when the Marine's arms are locked out. This procedure is repeated until the Marine has reached the maximum 20 complete pull-ups, or can no longer complete a pull-up.

- **Scoring:** The maximum number of correctly performed pull ups is recorded. Five points for every pull-up is awarded, and at least three are required to pass the test.
- **Comments:** Grip changes are allowed during the exercises, as long as the Marines feet do not touch the bars or ground, and his hands do not touch the side bars of the pull-up bar. Resting is allowed in the up or down position, but resting with the chin supported by the bar is not allowed. Sweat shirts need to be removed so that the locking of the elbows can be observed. Throughout the test, the legs may be in a straight or bent position, but may not be raised above the waist. Whipping, kicking, kipping of the body or legs, or any leg movement used to assist the pull-up is not allowed.

64

Punching Power Test

The Punching Power Test is part of the SPARQ rating system for boxing, and their protocol is listed here.

- **Purpose:** to measure maximal punching power
- **Equipment required:** instrumented 100-pound heavy punching bag, boxing gloves
- **Description / procedure:** A specially instrumented punching bag that can record the force of a hit is used. The athlete is allowed six maximal punches against the bag.
- **Scoring:** Peak and average punch power is recorded.
- **Target population:** boxing
- **Comments:** This test was used in the 3rd season of the Contender TV series to assess the fitness of the boxers.

65

Push - Up Test

This test measures upper body strength and endurance. The following information describes the procedures as used in the President's Challenge Fitness Awards.

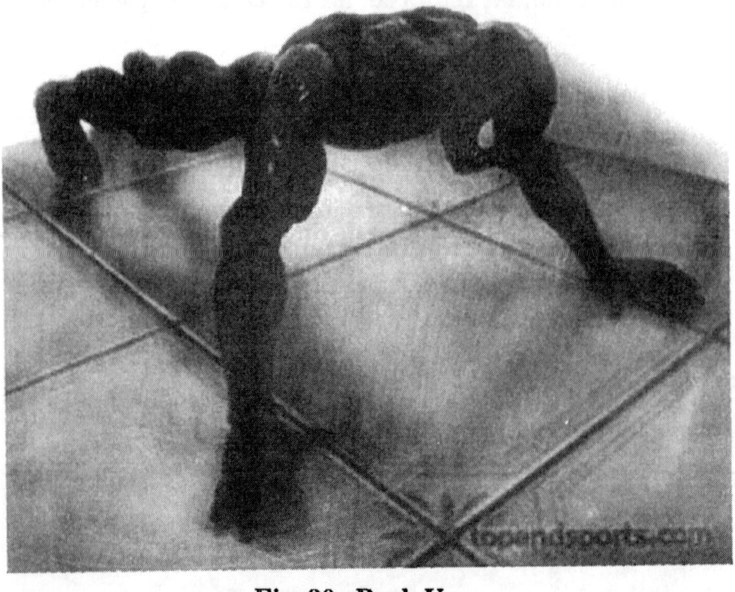

Fig. 30 : Push Up

- **Equipment required:** floor mat, metronome (or audio tape, clapping, drums)
- **Description / procedure:** Start in the push up position - with the hands and toes touching the floor, the body and legs are in a straight line, feet slightly apart, the arms at shoulder width apart, extended and at a right angles to the body. Keeping the back and knees straight, the subject lowers the body until there is a 90-degree angle at the elbows, with the upper arms parallel to the floor. A partner holds their hand at the point of the 90-degree angle so that the subject being tested goes down only until their shoulder touches the partner's hand, then back up. The push-ups are done in time to a metronome or similar device with one complete push-up every three seconds. The subject continues until the they can do no more in rhythm (has not done the last three in rhythm) or has reached the target number of push-ups.
- **Modifications:** Modifications of this test to make it easier, includes having the knees on the ground or to have the hands resting on a chair. Such modifications may be required when testing people with very weak upper body strength or females. Another modification is just to record the total number of push ups completed in a set time period or at any tempo.
- **Scoring:** Record the number of correctly completed push-ups that were performed in rhythm.
- **Target population:** sports in which upper body strength is important, such as rowing.
- **Advantages:** this test is easy and quick to perform.
- **Comments:** The subjects should be instructed to spend as little time in the starting position beforehand in order to reduce fatigue and increase the number of repetitions. The test is also sometimes called the press up test.

66

PWC-$_{170}$ Test & PWC$_{75\%}$ Tests

- **Purpose:** This test measures aerobic fitness
- **Comments:** PWC stands for physical work capacity. PWC-170 estimates the working capacity at a heart rate of 170 beats per minute, while PWC-75% estimates the working capacity at 75% of maximum heart rate. The procedures are very similar for the two tests, below is described the method for the PWC170. For the PWC75% the heart rates aim for each stage may be different.
- **Equipment required:** Cycle ergometer, clock or stopwatch, heart rate monitor (optional).
- **Description:** Athletes perform three consecutive workloads on a cycle ergometer. Begin by setting up subject on bike to ensure correct seat height (knee slightly bent at bottom of cycle). Place heart rate monitor on the subject. Check their exercise history to determine the starting workload (estimated to achieve a heart rate between 100-115). Start the test and measure heart rate each minute and continue for 3-4 minutes (until a steady heart rate is achieved). Continue the test for

2nd and 3rd workloads, set to achieve a HR between 115-130 and 130-145 beats per minute respectively.

- **Scoring:** Each steady-state heart rate and workload are graphed, with the line of best fit for the three points extrapolated to estimate the workload that would elicit a heart rate of 170 beats per minute (or 75% of maximum HR for the PWC-75% test). This workload value can then be compared to norms.
- **Validity:** Published research has shown a correlation between this test results and VO_{2max} scores of approximately 0.9.
- **Advantages:** The seated athlete makes it appropriate for ECG monitoring.
- **Disadvantages:** As it is performed on a cycle ergometer, the test favors cyclists. Determining the line of best fit and extrapolating to 170 bpm can be subjective and open to error.
- **Test versions:** As well as the PWC 170 and 75%, other levels may also be used, such as PWC 130 for measuring elderly or other populations in which you do not wish to excessively elevate the heart rate.
- **More information:** measuring heart rate

67

Quadrant Jump Test

- **Aim:** This is a whole body agility test, measuring the ability to move with maximum speed while maintaining balance and control (coordination).
- **Equipment required:** tape measure, chalk or tape for marking ground, stopwatch
- **Description / Procedure:** A quadrant is marked out on the floor, as illustrated in the diagram, with a starting line and numbered quadrants. The subject stands with both feet together at the starting line. On the command 'go', they jump ahead across the line into the first quadrant, then in sequence successively into quadrants 1, 2, 3, 4, 1, 2, etc. This pattern is continued as rapidly as possible for 10 seconds. After a rest repeat the trial.
- **Scoring:** The average score from two, 10 second trials is the subject's score.The subject's score is the number of correct jumps less a penalty deduction. One point is awarded each time the subject lands with both feet entirely within the correct quadrant during the 10 second trial, with a penalty of 0.5 point subtracted each time the subject touches a line and for each time the subject lands with one or both feet in an incorrect quadrant.

- **Advantages:** This is a simple agility test to perform, requiring limited equipment and space.
- **Disadvantages:** Only one person can perform the test at a time
- **Variations:** Comparison of performing the test in the anticlockwise and clockwise directions may show if any imbalances exist between left and right movement skills.

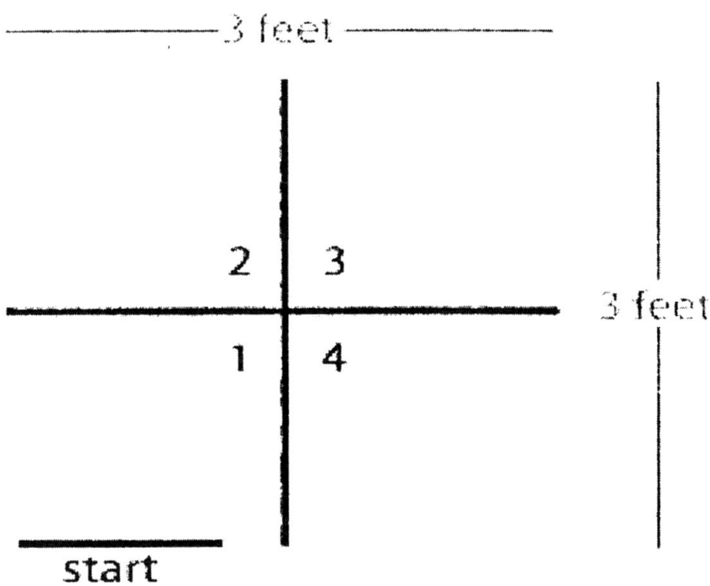

Fig. 31 : Quadrant Jump

68

Queens College Step Test

- **Purpose:** this step test provides a measure of cardio-respiratory or endurance fitness.
- **Equipment required:** 16.25 inches or 41.3 cm step, stopwatch, metronome or cadence tape, heart rate monitor (optional).
- **Description:** The athlete steps up and down on the platform at a rate of 22 steps per minute for females and at 24 steps per minute for males, for a total of 3 minutes. The athlete immediately stops on completion of the test, and the heart beats are counted for 15 seconds from 5-20 seconds of recovery.
- **Scoring:** an extimation of VO2max can be calculated form the test results, using the formula below:
  - Men: VO2max (ml/kg/min) = 111.33 - 0.42 x heart rate (bpm)
  - Women: VO2max (ml/kg/min) = 65.81 - 0.1847 x heart rate (bpm)
- **Reliability:** test re-test reliability for recovery heart rate was r = 0.92
- **Validity:** correlation between recovery heart rate and VO_{2max} was r = -0.75.

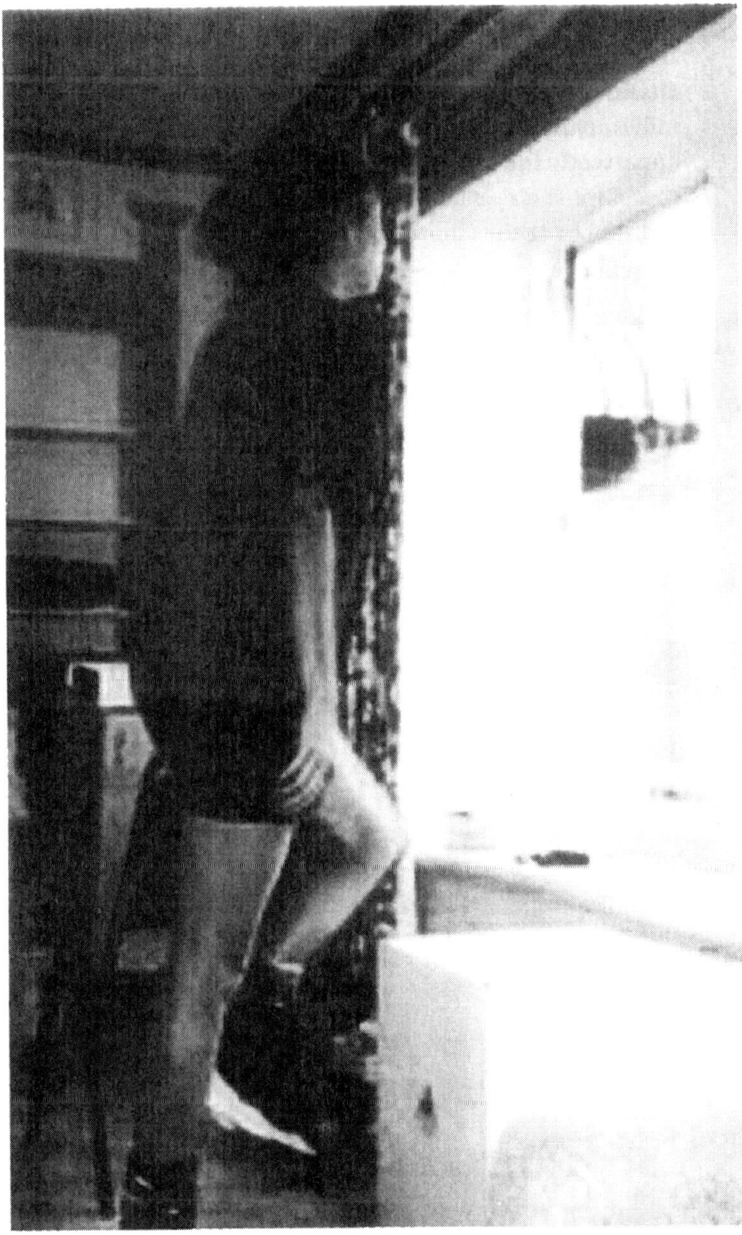

Fig. 32 : Queens College Step Test

- **Advantages:** minimal equipment and costs involved, little time required, and can be self-administered.
- **Disadvantages:** Biomechanical characteristics vary between individuals (e.g. taller people are at an advantage). Also, appartently the data was formulated from treadmill running, therefore their assumption is that stepping and treadmill running have the same oxygen cost.

69

Quick Strike Boxing Test

The Quick strike Test is part of the SPARQ rating system for boxing, and their protocol is listed here.

- **Purpose:** to measure sustained punching power
- **Equipment required:** instrumented 100-pound heavy bag, stopwatch, boxing gloves
- **Description / procedure:** This test utilizes a specially instrumented punching bag that can record the force and timing of a hit. The subject is instructed to hit the bag as fast and as hard as possible for a set time period.
- **Scoring:** the results include measures of peak punch and striking output
- **Target population:** boxing
- **Comments:** Strong verbal encouragement will help the subject achieve their maximal score. This test was used in the 3rd season of the Contender TV series to assess the fitness of the boxers.

70

Radar to Measure Speed

- **Purpose:** to measure peak speed of an object
- **Equipment required:** Radar Device. These can range in price from a few hundred dollars to thousands
- **Description / procedure:** A radar gun uses the Doppler Effect to detect the speed of objects. It transmits electromagnetic waves, which bounce off the object it is pointed at, returning to the device at a slightly different frequency. The radar detects the change in frequency, then computes this into a speed measurement. The radar can be set to record peak velocity, of either an object such as a ball, or the arm or bat, which is handy for many sports. The radar can be hand-held or one that can be placed on a tripod or on the ground. To get correct speed gun readings most radar guns will need to be placed directly in the line of travel of the object to be clocked, otherwise only a component of the true speed will be measured.
- **Target population:** radar can be used to measure running speed in sprinters, throwing speed in sports such as baseball, cricket, softball, and in hitting sports such as Tennis (serve speed) and golf (swing speed) and hockey.

- **Limitations:** A radar gun does not return information regarding the object's position. Peak speed will only be measured if the radar is placed directly in line of the moving object.
- **Accuracy:** The resolution of each radar may vary, ranging from +/-0.1 mph to +/- 1.0 mph. The accuracy is difficult to determine, as it would require you to find a object of known speed to calibrate against.
- **Range:** The radar will vary in how far away you can use the instrument. Some will be able to measure a moving object from a mile away.

Comments: Radar is an acronym for RAdio Detection and Ranging. It was invented by Bryce K. Brown of Decatur Electronics in March 1954.

71

Reaction Light Board Test

The Light Board Test is part of the SPARQ rating system for boxing, and their protocol is listed here.

- **Purpose:** to measure reaction time, hand-eye quickness and coordination.
- **Equipment required:** Bosu™ ball, instrumented light board
- **Description / procedure:** The light board is constructed so that when active, the board displays a target light that moves to different cells across the board. The lights are located a different distances on lines radiating out from the center of the board. The athlete stands upon a Bosu ball and facing the light board. The light board is positioned so that the center is directly in front of the face. The athlete tries to press as many active lights as possible.
- **Scoring:** The score is the number of lights that are pressed during the test, out of a total possible of 90.
- **Target population:** boxing

Comments: This test was used in the 3rd season of the Contender TV series to assess the fitness of the boxers.

72

Stress Questionnaire for Athletes

- **Purpose:** this tool is for evaluating athlete recovery using a questionnaire. Adequate recovery is important to restore the body to the pre-exercise state and prepare for the next bout of exercise.
- **Equipment required:** The RESTQ manual and CD, computer
- **Description / procedure:** The RESTQ-Sport questionnaire measures stress and recovery rates in athletes. The manual gives the user the tools needed to measure and track an athlete's recovery. The CD includes a database and scoring program. You are able to create a database of both individuals and groups. There are two questionnaires (RESTQ-76 and REST-52), scoring keys and profile sheets for the questionnaires.
- **Interpretation:** the manual provides various examples, in the form of case studies, of how to interpret the data.
- **Target groups:** This test is suitable for sport participants of all levels. The questionnaire can be used for both applied work and research.

73

Walk Test

- **Description:** The purpose of this test is to walk as fast as possible for 1 mile. After you have completed the mile, immediately take your pulse rate. If you do not have a heart rate monitor, you can manually count the number of beats for 10 seconds, and then multiply that by 6 to get your minute heart rate. Note the time it took to complete the mile.
- **Scoring:** A VO_{2max} score can be calculated using the following equation:
  Females: VO_2 = 139.168 - (0.388 x age) - (0.077 x weight in lb.) - (3.265 x walk time in minutes) - (0.156 x heart rate).
  Males: add 6.318 to the equation for females above.
- **Equipment required:** stopwatch, smooth and level marked 1 mile track, paper and pencil, heart rate monitor (optional).
- **Target population:** Suitable for both males and females of poor fitness who would not be able to complete a similar distance run test.
- **Advantages:** minimal equipment and costs are required, and the test can be self-administered.
- **Disadvantages:** This test is too easy for highly fit people. Also, since you must walk as fast as possible, the accuracy of this test depends on your pacing ability and level of motivation.

74

Run Or Walk For Set Time Or Distance

There are quite a few variations of the walking or running test as a measure of aerobic fitness. Here is a general description of this type of test. For specific instructions for a particular walking or running test, see the tests listed in *Related Pages* below. Also see the comparison page for a overview of the walk and run tests.

- **Description / procedure:** There are several tests which involve running for a set time (e.g. 9, 10, 12 minutes) or a set distance (1 mile, 1.5 mile, 1200m), and the distance covered or time required being recorded. The time required for these tests normally range from 8 to 15 minutes, depending on the population being tested.
- **Modifications:** In addition to different times and distances used for this test, different exercise modes such as swimming can be used. There are a few standard variations of this test, see Related Pages below.
- **Scoring:** norms are available for many of these tests. It is important to compare results to normative tales that have the same test procedures and with a similar target group.
- **Target population:** This test can be modified to be suitable for most populations. For adults, the test should be at least

10 minutes to ensure the energy demands are primarily supplied by the aerobic system. Shorter runs are more suitable for children.

- **Equipment required:** oval or running track, marking cones, recording sheets, stopwatch.
- **Validity:** Published studies generally have a correlation of 0.65 or better for runs of greater than 9 minutes or a mile.
- **Reliability:** reliability would depend on practice and pacing strategies and motivation level. There should be good reliability if these issues are addressed.
- **Advantages:** large groups can be tested at once, and it is a very cheap and simple test to perform.
- **Disadvantages:** practice and pacing is required, and performance on this test can be affected greatly by motivation.

75

Sharkey (Forestry) Step Test

This test was developed to evaluate the aerobic fitness of US Forestry workers.

- **Aim:** the purpose of this test is to determine aerobic fitness using a simple test and minimal equipment.
- **Equipment required:** step or platform 40 cm (15.75 inches) for males and 33 cm (13 inches) for females, stopwatch, metronome or cadence tape, body weight scales.
- **Description / procedure:** Record body weight measurement in the clothing to be used for the test. The metronome is set at 90 beats per minute, to indicate the stepping rate of 22.5 steps per minute. The subject steps up and down on the step, leading with either leg. Males are to use a higher step than females. After five minutes of stepping, the subject sits down and a heart rate measurement is taken. Count the number of heart beats, starting from 15 seconds after completing the test, and stop counting 15 seconds later at 30 seconds post-exercise.
- **Scoring:** Age, post-exercise heart rate, and body weight are used to calculate maximal aerobic power, using a published table. This score can then be compared to a table of norms.

- **Advantages:** This simple test requires minimal equipment and costs, can be performed indoors or out. It is possible to self-administer this test.
- **Disadvantages:** some subjects may not have the fitness or coordination to maintain the required stepping rate.
- **Comments:** this test was developed by Dr. Brian J. Sharkey, originally for testing fire fighters. Sharkey is a physiologist at the Forest Service's Missoula Technology and Development Center in Montana. He also helped develop the Work Capacity or "Pack" Test, which requires those who work on fires to carry a 45-pound pack three miles in 45 minutes.

76

Side-Step Test

- **Equipment:** flat, non-slip floor, with line markings (can use masking tape), tape measure, stopwatch
- **Description / procedure:** Subject stands at a center line, then jumps 30cm to the side (e.g. right) and touches a line with the closest foot, jumps back to the center then jumps 30 cm to the other side, then back to the center. This is one complete cycle. The subject tries to complete as many cycles as possible in one minute.
- **Scoring:** One complete cycle is recorded as 1, and half a cycle as 0.5. The score is expressed as the number of repetitions in one minute. Some normative values are presented below.

Table 20 : Side Step Test

	Poor	*Fair*	*Average*	*Good*	*High*
Female	<33	34-37	38-41	42-45	46+
Male	<37	38-41	42-45	46-49	50+

- **Equipment required:** stopwatch, measuring tape, lines marked on ground.

77

Skinfold Measurement

- **Description / procedure:** Estimation of body fat by skinfold thickness measurement. Measurement can use from 3 to 9 different standard anatomical sites around the body. The right side is usually only measured (for consistency). The tester pinches the skin at the appropriate site to raise a double layer of skin and the underlying adipose tissue, but not the muscle. The calipers are then applied 1 cm below and at right angles to the pinch, and a reading taken two seconds later. The mean of two measurements should be taken. If the two measurements differ greatly, a third should then be done, then the median value taken.
- **The sites:** there are many common sites at which the skinfold pinch can be taken. For a description and photographs of these sites go here.
- **Results:** Because of the increased errors involved, it is usually not appropriate to convert skinfold measures to percentage body fat (%BF). It is best to use the sum of several sites to monitor and compare body fat measures. In order to satisfy those who want to calculate a percentage body fat measure, there is a sample of equations for calculating this here. Below is a table of general guidelines for using total sum of the seven

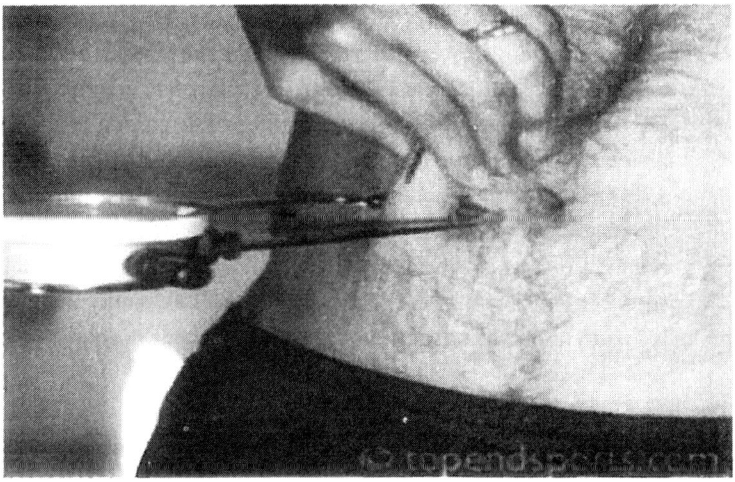

Fig. 33 : Hand Wall Toss Test Soon

main skinfold sites (tricep, bicep, subscap, supraspinale, abdominal, thigh, calf)

- **Equipment required:** skinfold calipers (e.g. Harpenden, Holtain, Slimglide, Lange). These should be calibrated for correct jaw tension and gap width.
- **Target population:** suitable for all populations, though it is sometimes difficult to get reliable measurements with obese people.
- **Validity :** using skinfold measurements is not a valid predictor of percent body fat, however they can be used as a monitoring device to indicate changes in body composition over time. It is important to maintain correct calibration of the calipers (more about calibrating calipers)
- **Reliability:** the reliability of skinfold measurements can vary from tester to tester depending on their skill and experience. There are accreditation courses available through ISAK.
- **Advantages:** Skinfold measurements are widely utilized to assess body composition. It is a lot simpler than hydrostatic weighing and many of the other body composition techniques. After the original outlay for calipers, the daily tests costs are minimal.

- **Other considerations:** some subjects may feel uncomfortable stripping down in front of the tester, therefore every effect should be made to make them feel comfortable. For legal reasons, it is wise to have another person present, and to have females testers for female subjects. The right side measurement is standard, though in some situations you may need to test someone on the left side. If so, you must record this and endeavor to always test on the same side for that person. Reasons for testing on the left side may include injuries, amputation, deformities, or other medical conditions.

78

Sprint Tests (30 Yards, 20m 30m, 40 Yards)

- **Purpose:** The purpose of this test is to determine acceleration, maximum running speed and speed endurance, depending on the distance run
- **Equipment required:** measuring tape or marked track, stopwatch or timing gates, cone markers.
- **Description / procedure:** The test involves running a single maximum sprint over a set distance, with time recorded. The test is conducted over different distances, such as 10, 20, 40 and/or 50 meters or yards, depending on the sport and what you are trying to measure. The starting position should be standardized, starting from a stationary position with a foot behind the starting line, with no rocking movements. If you have the equipment (e.g. timing gates), you can measure the time to run each split distances (e.g. 5, 10, 20 m) during the same run, and then acceleration and peak velocity can also be determined. It is usual to give the athletes an adequate warm-up and practice first, and some encouragement to continue running hard past the finish line.

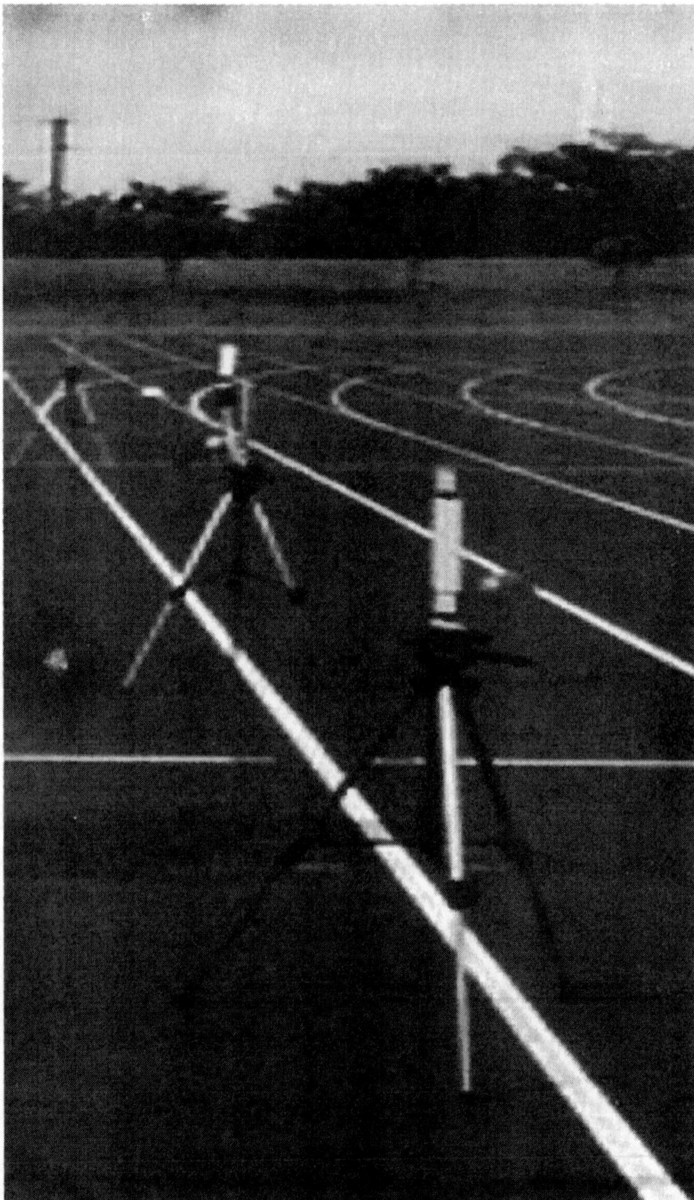

Fig. 34 : Spirit

Table 21 : Sprint Score

Time to run 35 meters (in seconds)

rating	*men*	*women*
very good	< 4.80	< 5.30
good	4.80 - 5.09	5.30 - 5.59
average	5.10 - 5.29	5.60 - 5.89
fair	5.30 - 5.60	5.90 - 6.20
poor	> 5.60	> 6.20

- **Results:** You can use a measure of the time for the first 10 meters or yards from a stationary start as a score for acceleration, and the time to run between 30-60 meters for a flying sprint speed, or maximum running speed. This score can also be presented as a running velocity (distance/ time). For sprint tests conducted over 100 meters or yards or so, comparing the time for the final 40 compared to the first 40 can be used as a speed endurance score.
- **Target population:** sprinters, team sport athletes.
- **Reliability:** Reliability is greatly improved if timing gates are used. Also weather conditions and running surface can affect the results, and these conditions should be recorded with the results. If possible, set up the track with a crosswind to minimize the effect of wind.

79

Fatigue Test

- **Purpose:** this is a test of anaerobic capacity, the ability to recover between sprints and produce the same level of power repeatedly.
- **Equipment required:** 2 stopwatches, measuring tape, marker cones, at least 50 meter track.
- **Description / procedure:** marker cones and lines are placed 30 meters apart to indicate the sprint distance. Two more cones placed a further 10 meters on each end. At the instructions of the timer, the subject places their foot at the starting line, then on 'go' two stopwatches are started simultaneously, and the subject sprints maximally for 30 m, ensuring that they do not slow down before reaching the end. One stopwatch is used to time the sprint, the other continues to run. Record the time. The subjects use the 10 meter cone to slow down and turn, and return to the 30 m finishing point. The next sprint will be in the oposite direction. The next 30 meter sprint starts 30 seconds after the first started. This cycle continues until 10 sprints are completed, starting at 30 sec, 1 min, 1.5 min, 2 min etc after the start of the first sprint.
- **Scoring:** The fatigue index is calculated by calculating the average speed of the first three trials and dividing it by the

average speed of the last three trials. This will give a value approximately between 75 and 95%. Use the table below to determine the rating.

Table 22 : Fatigue Index

Rating	*Fatigue Index*
Excellent	> 89%
Good	85-89 %
Average	80-84%
Poor	< 80%

- **Target population:** suitable for athletes involved in many multi-sprint sports such basketball, hockey, rugby, soccer.

80

Stress Test

An exercise stress test is commonly conducted by health professionals to determine cardiac function of people with heart disease risk factors.

- **Description / procedure:** A progressive and maximum exercise test (starting from a walking pace and gradually increasing pace) is performed while the electrical impulses from the heart tissue are recorded by surface electrodes places on the chest wall.
- **Equipment required:** Exercise machine such as a treadmill or exercise bike, a 12-lead ECG machine and leads, sticking tape, clips and other sundries as required.
- **Analysis**: Specialist training is required to interpret exercise ECG traces. Many of the stress testing machines can perform basic analysis, though these should not be relied on fully and a well trained human eye should look at the results before any conclusions are made.
- **Comments**: See your doctor is you think you need a stress test performed. A stress test can pick up early changes in the heart function indicating potential heart disease. The test is also known as a cardiac stress test.

- **Qualifications:** Stress tests are either performed by a medical practitioner, or a qualified health specialist with a doctor nearby.

81

Shuttle Swim Test

This test is a variation on the beep test, or shuttle run, called the Water Polo Intermittent Shuttle Test (WIST) or the 10 meter Multistage Shuttle Swim Test (MSST). This test has been developed by sport scientists in Western Australia, to assess a player's ability to perform repeated high-intensity efforts interspersed with brief periods of active recovery. Studies have found that it is a reliable and valid field test of aerobic fitness for use with trained water polo players.

- **Purpose:** To test the aerobic fitness of water polo players
- **Equipment required:** swimming pool, cd, cd player.
- **Description:** This test is a variation on the established testing protocol for the running shuttle test, but specific for water polo players and carried out in a pool. It is not continuous like the shuttle run — players swim, then rest, then swim, which replicates what would happen during a water polo game.
- **Scoring:** The athletes score is the level and number of shuttles reached before they were unable to keep up with the recording.
- **Target population:** It is a test of aerobic fitness for competitive water polo players. The test is suitable for all

players (male and female) ranging from school/club standard through to international level.

- **Reliability:** In the published research paper, test-retest reliability was determined using a sample of 22 female and 22 male water polo players. An intraclass correlation coefficient of 0.99 ($p>0.05$) was calculated between the two test scores. The technical error of measurement for the test was 2.3 shuttles or 5.0%.
- **Validity:** A validation correlation coefficient of 0.88 was found between the number of shuttles completed during the MSST and VO2max measured during an incremental tethered swim test to exhaustion. A stepwise multiple regression revealed that VO2max accounted for approximately 78% of the MSST variance.
- **Advantages:** The test allows a whole team to have their aerobic fitness effectively assessed using minimal time and pool space.
- **Disadvantages:** As with the running beep test, practice and motivation levels can influence the score attained, and the scoring can be subjective.
- **Comments:** The test was designed and produced by the Western Australian Institute of Sport and The University of Western Australia (Department of Human Movement and Exercise Science)

82

500yd / 450m Swim Test

This test is an alternative to the which forms part of the Navy Physical Readiness Test (PRT), performed by US Navy personnel every six months.

- **Purpose:** This test measures aerobic fitness and swimming ability.
- **Equipment required:** standard 25 or 50 yard/meter swimming pool, stopwatch
- **Description / procedure:** The aim of this test is to swim 500 yards or 450 meters in the fastest time possible. Any swim stroke and turn may be used. Swimmers begin the test in the water. On the command 'go,' the clock will start, and you will begin swimming at your own pace. The timer shall call out time intervals or lengths until completion of test. Swimmers may push off from sides with hands and feet after each pool length. Resting is permitted by holding side of pool, standing, or treading water. Swimmers may use goggles, face masks, swim caps, and or ear plugs, though fins, snorkels, flotation, wet suit, and propulsion devices are not allowed.
- **Scoring:** The total time to complete the distance is recorded, to the nearest second.

- **Comments:** the test will be stopped if the participant moves forward while resting, or receives or requires assistance from lifeguard or other person.

83

Body Electrical Conductivity (TOBEC)

- **Equipment required:** TOBEC device.
- **Method:** TOBEC is based on lean tissue being a better conductor of electricity than fat.
- **Description / procedure:** The subject lies in a cylinder that generates a very weak electromagnetic field. The strength of the field depends on the electrolytes found in the person's body water. In about 10 seconds, TOBEC makes 10 conductivity readings that estimate lean body mass.
- **Advantages:** very accurate noninvasive method for body composition analysis
- **Disadvantages:** equipment is costly.

84

Body Potassium (TBK)

- **Aim:** this procedure accurately determines the body's total cell mass (that is, the active growing tissues in the body), which in turn can be used to estimate fat-free or lean body mass. When this measurement is combined with measurements from the Total Body Protein, you can determine total organ and muscle mass.
- **Equipment required:** extremely sensitive equipment which measures the gamma rays emitted from the naturally occurring radioactive isotope of potassium known as 40K.
- **Description / procedure:** The subject must first be shielded from naturally occurring radiation in the environment, using concrete, lead or steel. Once the external radiation is minimized, the subject's natural radiation as 40K is measured through the use of scintillation counters. The radiated 40K is measured over a specified time period and from this TBK is estimated.
- **Advantages:** other than the initial outlay cost for equipment, this method is relatively simple to carry out, safe, and operational expenses are relatively small.

- **Disadvantages:** the required instrument is very expensive to install and has limited availability.
- **Comments:** The determination of TBK is based on the fact that the proportion of total potassium found in human tissues as 40K is constant at 0.0118% of total potassium. Therefore, by measuring 40K you can calculate total-body potassium. As potassium is distributed almost entirely within the intracellular compartment of fat-free mass, and using the ratio of total-body potassium to fat-free mass, once TBK is known you can calculate fat-free mass and total-body fat.
- **Use:** TBK is a classical method of quantifying total-body fat. It has mostly been replaced by newer more accurate techniques.

85

Body Protein (TBP)

- **Aim:** this technique measures the amount of nitrogen in the body, which is a direct indicator of total body protein (TBP).
- **Equipment required:** Prompt Gamma Activation Analyzer.
- **Description / procedure:** Before the scan begins, the subject undergoes measures of chest, arm, waist, and leg widths and thickness. These measurements are used to adjust the nitrogen scan data for a subject's size and shape. The subject then lies fairly still in the supine position as three separate body sections (legs, waist, chest) are measured for 10 minutes each. The scan involves irradiation of the subject with neutrons, and cause them to give off characteristic gamma rays. The gamma rays are collected from detectors placed on either side of the subject, and analyzed using conventional spectroscopy.
- **Results:** Total protein can be estimated from the ratio of nitrogen to hydrogen counts. Nitrogen and protein are closely linked with each other because of a stable chemical combination (protein is 16% nitrogen) and because over 98% of the total body nitrogen is in the form of protein.

- **Advantages:** When this measurement is combined with measurements from the Total Body Potassium Counter, it is possible to determine total organ and muscle mass.
- **Disadvantages:** the required instrument is very expensive to install and has limited availability.
- **Comments:** The system is called a *prompt gamma* system as the gammas are produced immediately, and stop appearing as soon as the neutron source is removed.
- **Use:** Prompt Gamma Activation Analysis is the gold-standard method for measuring the amount of nitrogen in the body, which in turn is a direct indicator of total body protein (TBP).

86

Aerobic Test

- **Equipment required:** Repco front access cycle ergometer (which uses air resistance to modify resistance), heart rate monitor (otherwise you can use the manual palpation method), work monitor unit (optional, some bikes have a workload dial attached to the cycle), stopwatch or clock, scales to determine the body weight of the athlete prior to the test.
- **Description / procedure:** The athlete pedals in one minute increments of 25 Watts (starting at 25 Watts) until their heart rate reaches 75% of their predicted maximum heart rate (estimated using the formula 220-age). They continue pedaling until the end of the minute during which the target heart rate is achieved. If the target heart rate is reached during the final minute, the workload at which it was achieved is calculated by extrapolation.
- **Scoring:** The workload at which the 75% predicted heart rate is achieved is recorded. This score is then divided by body weight (Aerobic Index), and norm tables are available for comparison to the general population.
- **Advantages:** The seated athlete makes it appropriate for ECG monitoring. This test suits older participants as it does not stress the body maximally.

- **Disadvantages:** As this test is performed on a cycle ergometer, it would favor cyclists.
- **More information:** measuring heart rate.

87

Rotation Test

The purpose of this flexibility test is to measure trunk and shoulder flexibility, which is important for injury prevention and in particular is important in swimming, racquet sports and throwing sports.

- **Equipment required:** wall, a piece of chalk or pencil, ruler or tape measure.
- **Description / procedure:** Mark a vertical line on the wall. Stand with your back to the wall directly in front of the line, with your feet shoulder width apart. You should be about arms length away from the wall, though you may need to adjust the distance from the wall once you start the test. Extend your arms out directly in front of you so they are parallel to the floor. Twist your trunk to your right and the touch the wall behind you with your fingertips, keeping your arms extended and parallel to the floor. You are allowed to turn your shoulders, hips and knees as long as your feet don't move. Mark the position where your fingertips touched the wall, and measure the distance from the line. A point before the line is a negative score and a point after the line is a positive score. Repeat for the left side with your feet in the same position.

- **Scoring:** Take the average of the 2 scores (left and right sides). Use the table below to convert the score measurement to a rating.
- **Aadvantages:** simple and quick test to perform. Athletes can perform the test themselves.
- **Disadvantages:** Variations in arm length between individuals may make comparisons more difficult.

88

T-Test

- **Purpose:** the T-Test is a test of agility for athletes, and includes forward, lateral, and backward running.
- **Equipment required:** tape measure, marking cones, stopwatch, timing gates (optional).
- **Description / Procedure:** Set out four cones as illustrated in the diagram above. The subject starts at cone A. On the command of the timer, the subject sprints to cone B and touches the base of the cone with their right hand. They then turn left and shuffle sideways to cone C, and also touches its base, this time with their left hand. Then shuffling sideways to the right to cone D and touching the base with the right hand. They then shuffle back to cone B touching with the left hand, and run backwards to cone A. The stopwatch is stopped as they pass cone A.
- **Scoring:** The trial will not be counted if the subject cross one foot in front of the other while shuffling, fails to touch the base of the cones, or fails to face forward throughout the test. Take the best time of three successful trials to the nearest 0.1 seconds. The table below shows some scores for adult team sport athletes.

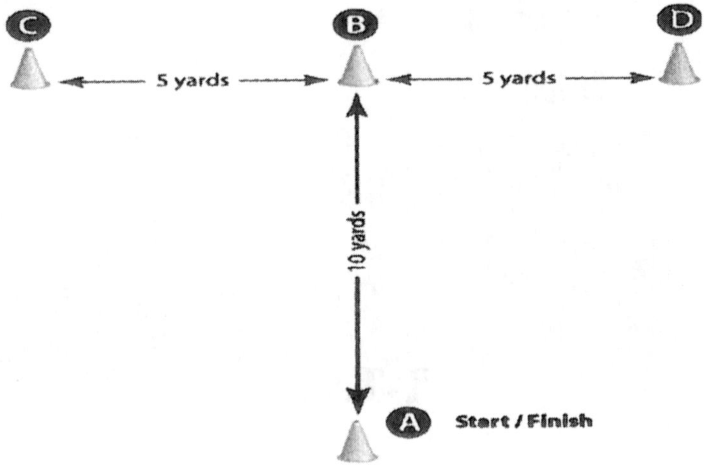

Fig. 35 : T-Test

- **Comments:** Ensure that the subjects face forwards when shuffling and do not cross the feet over one another. For safety, a spotter should be positioned a few meters behind cone A to catch players in case they fall while running backward through the finish.
- **Reliability:** the type of surface that is used should be consistent to ensure good test-retest reliability.
- **Advantages:** This is a simple agility test to perform, requiring limited equipment and space.
- **Disadvantages:** Only one person can perform the test at a time.

Table 23 : T-less Scores

	Males (seconds)	*Females (seconds)*
Excellent	< 9.5	< 10.5
Good	9.5 to 10.5	10.5 to 11.5
Average	10.5 to 11.5	11.5 to 12.5
Poor	> 11.5	> 12.5

89

Lung Function - Peak Flow

- **Description / procedure:** First make sure you have no food or gum in your mouth and stand up. Put the pointer on the gauge of the peak flow meter at 0. Attach the mouthpiece to the peak flow meter. Take a deep breath, then place the peak flow meter mouthpiece in your mouth and close your lips tightly around the outside of the mouthpiece (don't put your tongue inside the mouthpiece). Breathe out as hard and as fast as possible (using a "huff" rather than a full breath out). Record the value on the gauge before moving the pointer on the gauge back to 0. At least three attempts should be performed.
- **Equipment required:** peak flow meter, which can come as a small pocket-sized machine.
- **Results:** Record the highest value of all attempts. The value recorded is peak expiratory flow (PEF), in liters per minute.
- **Comments:** as PEF results depend on how hard you try, it is very important to blow as hard and fast as possible, and to take as many attempts as necessary to get the best result. As only peak flow is measured, which occurs during the first part of expiration, it is not necessary to expel all the air form the lungs at each attempt. People who use a home peak flow

meter need to use the same meter over time because different brands of meters may give different values for results. If you change meters, you need to determine your personal best measurement using the new machine. Wash meters in soapy water every 2 weeks to prevent growth of bacteria.

- **Interpretation:** Lung function tests are of little value for predicting fitness and exercise performance, provided that the values fall within a normal range. Peak flow is used as an indicator of asthma or similar.
- **Advantages:** small portable and inexpensive peak flow meters are available that are great for the asthmatic to monitor their own lung function at any time.
- **Disadvantages:** Peak expiratory flow meter results are not as accurate as lung function measures through spirometry.

90

Jump by Measuring Jump Time

Vertical jumping ability is important for many sports, and there are a plethora of programs for training to increase your vertical jump ability. It is important to monitor the changes in your vertical jump, to see if there really are increases. The traditional method for assessing vertical jump ability is by measuring jump height using a wall or Vertec device. The method described below measures the jump air time using an electrical contact operated systems, and from that calculates jump height. This is the preferred method when testing for the SPARQ rating system.

- **Equipment required:** Electronic timing mat, such as the Just Jump System, or infrared laser system
- **Description / procedure:** Jump height can be calculated using a timing mat or laser system which measures the time the feet are off the mat. The athlete stands as still as possible on the mat with weight evenly distributed over both feet. Once the mat is reset, the athlete jumps vertically as high as possible using both arms and legs to assist in projecting the body upwards. The athlete then lands back on the mat with both feet landing at the same time. A score of the time in the air, and the calculated vertical jump height is then given.

Height can be calculated using this formula: jump height = 4.9 x (0.5 x Time)^2). The best score of at least three attempts is recorded.

- **Variations:** Vertical jump height can also be measured using a Vertec or wall. Other test modifications are to perform the test with no arm movement (one hand on hip, the other raised above the head) to isolate the leg muscles and reduce the effect of variations in coordination of the arm movements. The vertical jump test is usually performed with a countermovement, that is, there is bending of the knees prior to the vertical jump. The test can also be performed as a squat jump, starting from the position of knees being bent, say at 90 degrees. The test can also be performed off one leg, with a single step into the jump, or with a run-up, depending on the relevance to the sport involved.
- **Scoring:** The jump height Jump is usually recorded as the score in distance. The table below provides a ranking scale for adult athletes based on my observations, and will give a general idea of what is a good score. For more information, see a selection of vertical jump test results.

There are also a calculation to convert jump height into a power or work score. Here are several formula I have come across.

- Power = 2.21 x weight x root of jump distance.
- Power = body mass(kg) x (4.9 x height jumped in meters)^2
- Peak Anaerobic Power output (Watts)

PAPw = (60.7 x jump height) + (45.3 x body mass(kg) - 2055)

- **Advantages:** this test is simple and quick to perform. This jump timing mat device is very portable, compared to the Vertec, though the laser system is more bulky and expensive. The vertical jump measurement when using this device is also not reliant on the subject timing their jump to touch something at the peak of the jump. Many timing mats can also be used for timing sprints and other uses.
- **Disadvantages:** To be accurate, you must ensure that both feet land back on the mat with legs nearly fully extended, as

Table 24 : Jump Height Power Conversion

Rating	*Males (inches)*	*Males (cm)*	*Females (inches)*	*Females (cm)*
excellent	> 28	> 70	> 24	> 60
very good	24 - 28	61-70	20 - 24	51-60
above average	20 - 24	51-60	16 - 20	41-50
average	16 - 20	41-50	12 - 16	31-40
below average	12 - 16	31-40	8 - 12	21-30
poor	8 - 12	21-30	4 - 8	11-20
very poor	< 8	< 21	< 4	< 11

landing with the legs bent can give incorrect larger scores. Without a mark on the wall to aim for and motivate the subject, measured jump height using this method is often lower than other methods. As the mat responds to the movement of weight on and off the mat, they are sometimes too sensitive and give erroneous results or are hard to stabilize before starting the test. This mats can be quite expensive.

- **Comments:** The jump height can be affected by how much you bend your knees before jumping, and the effective use of the arms. As with many tests, motivation can affect results - you should provide encouragement to the participant to achieve their maximal score.

91

Colour Measurement

- **Description / procedure:** The first part of the urine stream is discarded, then a small sample of urine is collected into a clear container. Measurement may be done immediately, or the specimen can be stored for later analysis. The sample is usually collected first thing in the morning. It may also be of interest to collect samples prior to or post exercise, though there may be a time delay for the effect of dehydration to show in the urine color.
- **Equipment required:** Urine specimen containers, ice bucket for storage and ice, color rating chart, gloves, clip boards, recording sheet, pen.
- **Interpretation:** The sample should be held up in front of a white background, in good light, and the color compared to the chart to the left. The lower the number, the better the result. A urine color rating of 1, 2 or 3 is considered to be well-hydrated (Armstrong, 2000). Based on these results, changes in fluid intake can be made.
- **Precautions**:
    - certain medicines and vitamins may cause the color of the urine to change. If any of these have been taken, this test is unreliable.

- sthe colors your see on the screen, or when you print the image out, may appear different to the original chart. Therefore this chart should only be used as a guide. If more accurate comparison is required, please go to an original source.

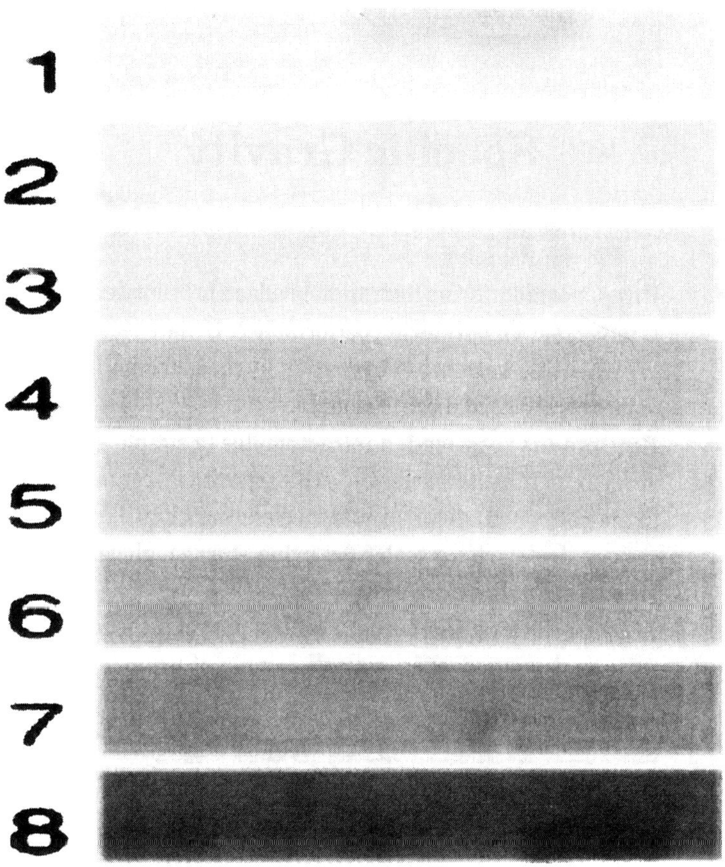

Fig. 36 : Colour Rating Chart

92

Specific Gravity

- **Purpose:** monitoring hydration levels to prevent dehydration is important for optimizing performance. Urine specific gravity is a scientific measure of hydration by measuring the density (concentration) of a urine sample.
- **Equipment required:** a refractometer (a simple hand-held version is illustrated here), urine specimen containers for urine collection, distilled water, cleaning cloth / disposable tissues, fridge or ice cooler for urine storage, gloves.
- **Description / procedure:**

1. **Collecting the urine.** The first part of the urine stream is discarded, then a small sample of urine is collected into a container. The sample can be measured immediately or stored for later measurement.
2. **Calibrating the refractometer.** Calibrate the refractometer by placing distilled water on the glass as the sample, and adjusting the scale to read 1.000. This should be done before you begin testing, and after every ten samples or so to ensure that the calibration remains accurate.
3. **Measurement.** Open up the flap at the end of the refractometer. Clean with distilled water and dry with a soft non-abrasive cloth. Place a drop of urine on the

glass plate and close the flap. Hold the refractometer up towards an area of natural light, look though the eye piece and read the specific gravity level off the scale - the point where the contrast line (difference between light and dark areas) crosses the scale.

4. **Results:** The measurement may be done immediately after collection, or the specimen can be stored in refrigeration for later analysis. The specific gravity results will range from 1.000 (which is equivalent to water) up to 1.035 (very dehydrated). There are several levels that are used in the literature to indicate dehydration, such as a value of 1.15 or greater.

- **Comments:** The sample is usually collected first thing in the morning. It may also be of interest to collect samples prior to or post exercise, though there may be a time delay for the effect of dehydration to show in the specific gravity measure.
- **Precautions:** certain medicines, vitamins or the presence of glucose may cause the urine specific gravity to change and give incorrect readings of dehydration. If any of these situations occur then the test is unreliable. The refractometer should be calibrated before you begin testing, and after every ten samples or so to ensure that the calibration remains accurate.
- **Advantages:** The hand held refractometer is very easy to operate.
- **Disadvantages:** This test requires the collection of urine (which is sometimes difficult) and the purchase of a specific apparatus for measurement. For a more simple test of hydration you can use urine color.

93

Waist to Hip Ratio

Aim: The purpose of this test to determine the ratio of waist circumference to the hip circumference, as this has been shown to be related to the risk of coronary heart disease.

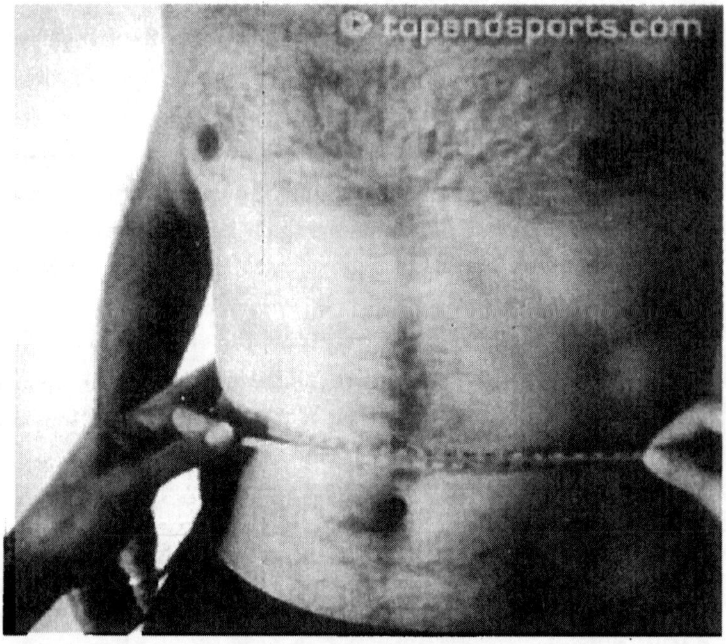

Fig. 37 : Waist to Hip

Table 25 : Waist to Hip Ratio

	Acceptable		*Unacceptable*		
	excellent	good	average	high	extreme
male	< 0.85	0.85 - 0.90	0.90 - 0.95	0.95 - 1.00	> 1.00
female	< 0.75	0.75 - 0.80	0.80 - 0.85	0.85 - 0.90	> 0.90

- **scoring:** The table below gives general guidelines for acceptable levels for hip to waist ratio. You can use any units for the measurements (e.g. cm or inches), as it is only the ratio that is important.
- **Equipment required:** tape measure
- **Description / procedure:** A simple calculation of the measurements of the waist girth divided by the hip girth. Waist to Hip Ratio (WHR) = Gw / Gh, where Gw = waist girth, Gh = hip girth
- **Target population:** This measure is often used to determine the coronary artery disease risk factor associated with obesity.
- **Advantages:** the WHR is a simple measure that can be taken at home by anyone to monitor their own body composition levels.
- **Other comments:** The basis of this measure as a coronary disease risk factor is the assumption is that fat stored around the waist poses a greater risk to health than fat stored elsewhere in the body.

94

2 Km Walk Test

- **Equipment required:** stopwatch, marked 2 km track or path on level ground with firm and smooth surface, heart rate monitor (optional).
- **Description:** The test involves a brisk walking performance accompanied by simple measurements. It provides direct information on walking fitness (time and heart rate) and can be used to predict maximal oxygen uptake.
- **Scoring:** The results are calculated from the time of the 2 km walk, heart rate at the end of the walk, body mass index and age. Norms are available to place individual scores within a fitness category.
- **Target population:** Adults aged 20-65 of poor fitness who would not be able to complete a running test.
- **Reliability:** good, except with people with a high VO_{2max}.
- **Advantages:** minimal equipment and costs involved, can be self-administered or large groups at once.

- **Disadvantages:** this test is too easy for the highly fit person. One o fthe other running tests would be better suited.

95

Lung Function Testing

- **Description / procedure:** The usual measures of lung function are of forced vital capacity (FVC) and forced expired volume in 1 second (FEV_1). These can be measured with a full maximal expiration. Explain to the subject that they must fill their lungs completely, seal their lips around the mouthpiece, and empty their lungs as hard and fast as possible. The best of two trials is usually recorded.
- **Equipment required:** Spirometer (e.g. Vitalograph)
- **Interpretation:** Lung function tests are of little value for predicting fitness and exercise performance, provided that the values fall within a normal range. You must always take into consideration that lung volumes vary with age, sex and body size (especially height).
- **Disadvantages:** this test requires expensive equipment that is not always available. A simple inexpensive measure of lung function is the peak flow test.

96

Sit Test

- **Purpose:** The Wall Sit test is a measure of lower body strength endurance, particularly the quadriceps muscle.
- **Equipment required:** smooth wall and a stopwatch.

Table 26 : Wall Sit Score

Rating	*Males (seconds)*	*Females (seconds)*
excellent	>100	> 60
good	75 100	45-60
average	50-75	35-45
below average	25-50	20-35
very poor	< 25	< 20

- **Description / procedure:** Stand comfortably with feet approximately shoulder width apart, with your back against a smooth wall. Slowly slide your back down the wall to assume a position with both your knees and hips at a 90° angle. The timing starts when one foot is lifted off the ground and is stopped when the subject cannot maintain the position and the foot is returned to the ground. After a period of rest, the other leg is tested.

- **Scoring:** the total time in seconds that the position was held for each leg is recorded. The table below gives a general guideline to expected scores for adults, based on my personal experiences.
- **Advantages:** This test requires minimal equipment and can be conducted with large groups all at once.

97

Field Test (MFT) For Wheelchair Users

- **Purpose:** This test is a wheelchair version of the beep test, developed to evaluate physical fitness and predict peak oxygen consumption of wheelchair users.
- **Equipment required:** audio recording, cones, flat hard surface.
- **Description:** An octagonal course is marked out using cones. The course is basically a 15 m x 15 m square, with each corner modified to create a 2.83 m long turning zone. The four main sides of the octagon are 11 m long. The corner zones avoid the necessity to make a sharp 90 degree turn. The initial wheeling velocity is 6 km/hr, which increased by 0.37 km/hr in one minute stages. A beep signified when the subject had to be within the turning zone. The test was stopped if the subject was unable to reach the turning zone on three consecutive occasions.
- **Scoring:** The score is the number of exercise level achieved before they were unable to keep up with the recording.
- **Target population:** It is a test of aerobic fitness for people in wheel chairs.
- **Comments:** The subjects are allowed to use their own personal wheelchair and are free to choose the direction of

rotation for the test (clockwise or counterclockwise). It is also possible to simultaneously test four subjects if they choose the same direction of rotation for the test.

- **Advantages:** this test is more cost-effective and easier to administer than the alternative laboratory fitness tests that are usually required to test the fitness of wheelchair users.
- **Disadvantages:** As with the running beep test, practice and motivation levels can influence the score attained, and the scoring can be subjective. Wheelchair skill and technique may also affect the level achieved.

98

Yo -Yo Intermittent Recovery Test

The Yo-Yo Intermittent Test is similar to the Yo-Yo endurance test (a variation of the beep test), except in the intermittent tests the participants have a short active break (5 and 10 seconds for the endurance and recovery test, respectively).

- **Purpose:** The test evaluates an individual's ability to repeatedly perform intervals over a prolonged period of time, particularly for athletes from sports such as tennis, team handball, basketball and soccer.
- **Diagram:**

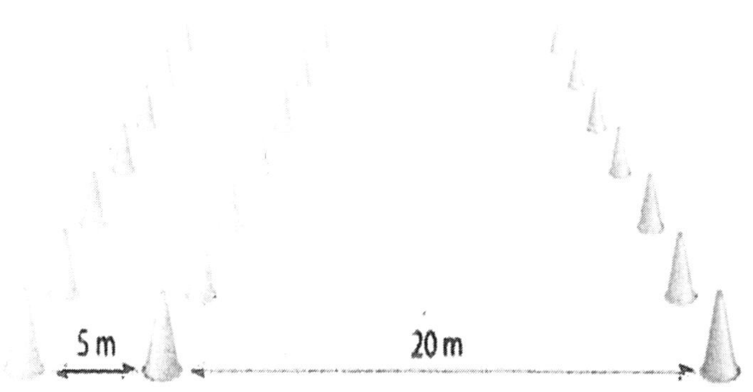

Fig. 38 : Marking Cones -7

- **Equipment required:** Flat, non-slip surface, marking cones, measuring tape, pre-recorded audio cassette or cd, cd or cassette player, recording sheets.
- **Description:** Use cones to mark out three lines as per the diagram above; 20 meters and 5 meters apart. The subject starts on or behind the middle line, and begins running 20 m when instructed by the cd. This subject turns and returns to the starting point when signaled by the recorded beep. There is a active recovery period (5 and 10 seconds respectively for the endurance and recovery versions of the test) interjected between every 20 meter (out and back) shuttle, during which the subject must walk or jog around the other cone and return to the starting point. A warning is given when the subject does not complete a successful out and back shuttle in the allocated time, the subject is removed the next time they do not complete a successful shuttle.
- **Variations:** There are two test levels: the Yo-Yo test level 1 test (designed for lesser trained individuals) starts at 10 km/hr and level 2 test (aimed at well trained and elite athletes) starts at 13 km/hr, with both levels increasing in speed throughout the test.
- **Scoring:** The athlete's score is the total distance covered before they were unable to keep up with the recording. The Yo-Yo intermittent test usually takes between 6-20 minutes for level 1 and between 2-10 minutes for level 2. See some Yo Yo Test Results.
- **Target population:** This test is suitable for sports teams and school groups, but not for populations in which a maximal exercise test would be contraindicated.
- **Reliability:** Reliability would depend on how strictly the test is run, and the previous practice allowed for the subjects.
- **Advantages:** Large groups can perform this test all at once for minimal costs.
- **Disadvantages:** Practice and motivation levels can influence the score attained, and the scoring of when a person is out of the test can be subjective. As the test is usually conducted outside, the environmental conditions can also affect the results.

- **Other considerations:** This test is a maximal test, which requires a reasonable level of fitness. It is not recommended for recreational athletes or people with health problems, injuries or low fitness levels.

99

Zig - Zag Test

- **Equipment required:** marker cones, stopwatch, non-slip surface.

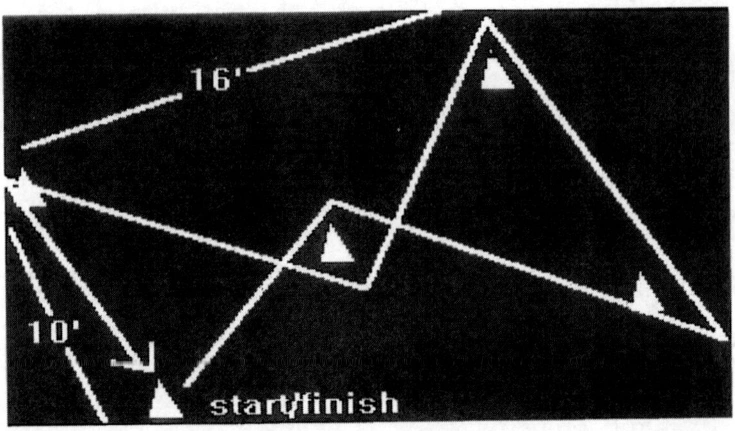

Fig. 39 : Zig-Zag Test

- **Description / procedure:** Similar to the Shuttle Run test, this test requires the athlete to run a course in the shortest possible time. A standard zig zag course is with four cones placed on the corners of a rectangle 10 by 16 feet, with one more cone placed in the centre. If the cones are labelled 1 to 4 around the rectangle going along the longer side first, and the centre cone is C, the test begins at 1, then to C, 2, 3, C, 4, then back to 1.

- **Modifications:** This test procedure can be modified by changing the distance between cones, and the number of circuits performed.
- **Comments:**The total distance run should not be too great so that fatigue does not become a factor.

100

Standing Stork Test

Objective

To monitor the development of the athlete's ability to maintain a state of equilibrium (balance) in a static position.

Required Resources

To undertake this test you will require:

Warm dry location - gym

Stop watch

How to conduct the test

Stand comfortable on both feet

Hands on your hip

Lift one leg and place the toes of that foot against the knee of the other leg

On command from the coach:

Raise the heel and stand on your toes

Coach starts the stop watch

Balance for as long as possible without letting either the heel touch the ground or the other foot move away from the knee.

Coach records the time you were able to maintain the balance

Repeat the test for the other leg.

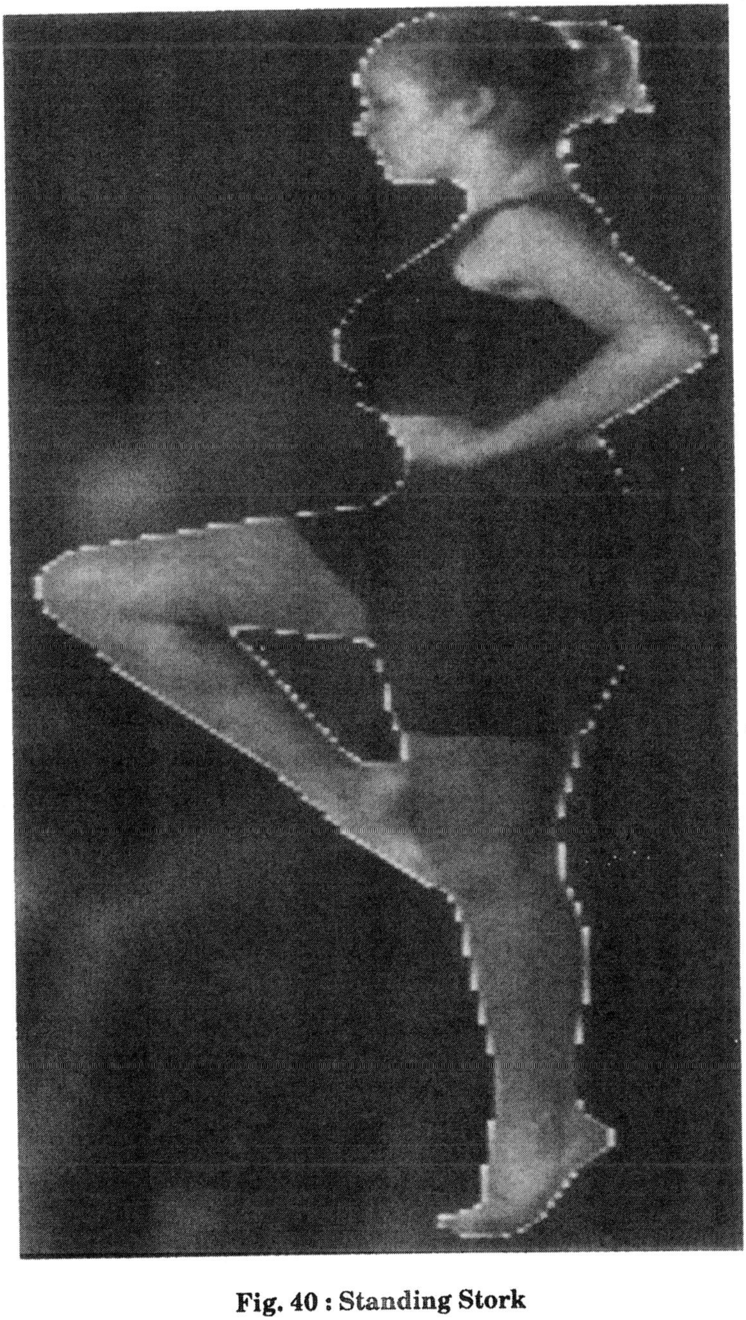

Fig. 40 : Standing Stork

Performance Assessment

For an evaluation of a 16 to 19 year old athlete's performance select the gender, enter the total time and then select the 'Calculate' button.

Normative data for the Stork Test

The following are national norms for 16 to 19 year olds.

Table 27 : Stork Test

Gender	*Excellent*	*Above Average*	*Average*	*Below Average*	*Poor*
Male	>50 secs	50 - 41 secs	40 - 31 secs	30 - 20 secs	<20 secs
Female	>30 secs	30 - 23 secs	22 - 16 secs	15 - 10 secs	<10 secs

Table Reference: Arnot R and Gaines C, Sports Talent, 1984.

101

NCF Abdominal Curl Conditioning Test

Objective

The objective of the NCF Abdominal Curl Conditioning Tests is to monitor the condition and tone of the athlete's abdominal muscles.

Required Resources

To undertake this test you will require:

Gym mat

NCF Abdominal Curl Conditioning Test audio tape or CD

Tape recorder or CD Player

Stop watch

Assistant

The NCF Abdominal Curl Conditioning Test audio tape or CD can be purchased from Coachwise 1st4Sport.

How to conduct the test

Follow the instructions on the tape or CD. Athletes are required to perform as many sit ups as possible, keeping in time to the beeps emitted from the tape or CD. The assistant counts the number of sit ups completed correctly and records the time from the start of the test until the athlete can no longer keep in time with the beeps or when the sit ups are not performed correctly.

Analysis

Analysis of the result is by comparing it with the results of previous tests. It is expected that, with appropriate training between each test, the analysis would indicate an improvement.

Performance Assessment

Normative scores

Table 28 : Conditioning Test Score

Stage	*Number of sit ups Cumulative*	*Standard Male*	*Standard Female*
1	20	Poor	Poor
2	42	Poor	Fair
3	64	Fair	Fair
4	89	Fair	Good
5	116	Good	Good
6	146	Good	Very Good
7	180	Excellent	Excellent
8	217	Excellent	Excellent

Notes

A degree of caution is required in administering the test, in that you have to push yourself relatively hard to the point where you can no longer maintain the pace dictated by the tape or CD. If you are suffering from any injury or illness, or if you have any reason to think you may not be in a good general state of health, you should consult a doctor before doing this test.

As the audio-tapes may stretch over time, the tapes need to be calibrated which involves timing a one-minute interval and making adjustment to the distance between markers. The recording is also available on compact disc, which does not require calibration.

102

Anaerobic Threshold Testing

The most accurate method of determining your Anaerobic Threshold (AT) is to visit a one of a number of establishments who can carry out a test under laboratory conditions. This generally costs money and usually means regular blood samples are taken to measure the amount of lactate in the blood during the workout. It is also likely that whilst undergoing this test your VO2 maximum and maximum heart rate will also be tested.

As this type of test is not readily available for all of us, the threshold can be discovered in other ways. The methods described below should not be taken as being very accurate in themselves, as not all the tests suit every one, but can be treated as excellent indicators. In all cases, a monitor that is capable of recording your heart rate is essential.

Threshold Testing

10km run

One method of finding your threshold is to complete a 10km race. Often this distance is run at around the threshold heart rate. You will need to record your heart rate as often as possible and the mile splits. If you are fit you will run fast and hard and achieve a constant heart rate. For those who are not so fit or start to fast the chances are you will at some point run above your threshold. This is usually followed by a dramatic drop in heart rate as you recover from the build up of excess lactic acid and a rise in the rate of respiration followed by a drop in pace. Sometimes this is accompanied by a burning sensation in the legs. If you notice these signs whilst running then check your monitor as there is a good chance that you have discovered your threshold. A 10km race can of course be simulated in training. Remember to rest the day before and take it easy for a couple of days after.

Per cent of MHR

One other method is to take an educated guess based on an assumption that your AT falls between 85 to 90% of your maximum heart rate (MHR)

Threshold Training

Having discovered your threshold it is important to work on improving it. You can start with one or two 6 to 10 minute repetitions building towards a sustained twenty minute run. As you become fitter so more 10 minute repetitions can be added to your schedule - say up to six. Your heart rate should be set at around 5% below your known threshold. These sessions should be run up to twice a week before peaking for a race season and once a week or less during the endurance build up - it is dependant upon your experience and fitness. These hard threshold runs should be preceded and followed by a recovery run. It is worth recording, charting and analysing all threshold runs. It is advisable to check your threshold every eight to six weeks.

103

Static Flexibility Test - Ankle

Objective

The objective of this test is to monitor the development of the athlete's Ankle flexibility.

How to conduct the test

Starting position

- Stand facing a wall
- Feet flat on the ground toes touching the wall
- Lean into the wall

Movement

- Slowly slide the feet back from the wall as far as possible
- Keep the feet flat on the ground, body and knees fully extended and the chest in contact with the wall
- Measure the distance between the toe line and the wall - to the nearest 1/4 of an inch
- Repeat the test 3 times and record the best distance

Analysis

Analysis of the result is by comparing it with the results of previous tests. It is expected that, with appropriate training between each test, the analysis would indicate an improvement.

Top of Form

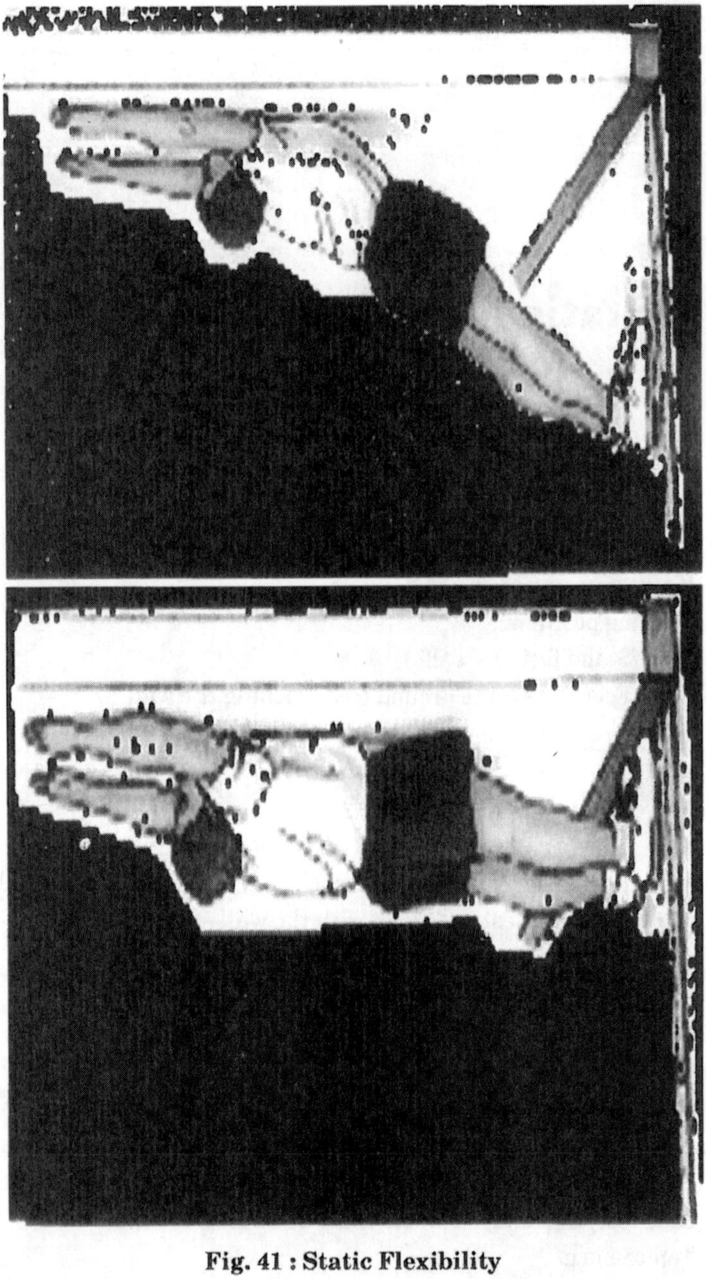

Fig. 41 : Static Flexibility

Performance Assessment

For an evaluation of the athlete's performance select the gender, enter the distance and then select the 'Calculate' button.

Normative data for the ankle flexibility test

Measurements are in inches.

Table 29 : Ankle Flexibility Score

Rating	*Men*	*Women*
Excellent	>35.00	>32.00
Good	35.00 - 32.51	32.00 - 30.51
Average	32.50 - 29.51	30.50 - 26.51
Fair	29.50 - 26.50	26.50 - 24.25
Poor	<26.50	<24.25

Table adapted from Johnson B.L. & Nelson J.K. Practical Measurements for Evaluation in PE 4th Ed. 1986

104

Astrand Treadmill Test

Objective

To monitor the development of the athlete's general endurance (VO2 max).

Required Resources

To undertake this test you will require:

- Treadmill where the speed can be set at 5 mph (8.05 km/hr) and grade of slope can be adjusted
- Stopwatch
- An assistant

How to conduct the test

The treadmill is set up at the start with a speed of 8.05 km/hr (5 mph) and a grade of slope of 0%. The athlete commences the test. After 3 minutes, the grade is set to 2.5% (1.4°) and then every 2 minutes the grade is increased by 2.5% (1.4°).

The assistant starts the stopwatch at the start of the test and stops it when the athlete is unable to continue.

Analysis of the test result

Analysis of the result is by comparing it with the results of previous tests. It is expected that, with appropriate training between each test, the analysis would indicate an improvement.

From the total running time an estimate of the athlete's VO2max can be calculated as follows:

VO2 max=(Time × 1.444) + 14.99

"Time" is the total time of the test expressed in minutes and fractions of a minute.

Example

The athlete stopped the test after 13 minutes 15 seconds of running (13.25 minutes).

- VO2 max=(13.25 × 1.444) + 14.99
- Vo2 max=34.123 mls/kg/min

105

Astrand 6 Minute Cycle Test

Objective

The objective of this test is to monitor the athlete's Vo2 max.

Required Resources

To undertake this test you will require:

- Cycle ergometer
- Heart rate monitor
- Stop watch
- An assistant

How to conduct the test

- Set up the cycle ergometer with correct handlebar and seat adjustments
- Select a load to begin the test - see the Astrand Test Loading Wattages table below. Whether you use the lower or upper wattages will depend upon your weight and fitness level. The selected load should raise your pulse rate to steady state between 130-160 bpm.
- Pedal at 60 rpm for 6 minutes at your chosen loading, taking pulse every minute. Your pulse rate should be steady state between 130-160 bpm

Table : 30 Astrand Test Loading Wattages

Age years	*Males*	*Females*
Under 35	100-150	100-125
35-55	100-125	75-100
Over 55	75-100	50-75

- If your pulse rate is not in the target range after 2 minutes then adjust your loading accordingly by 25 watts for the remainder of the test
- At the end of minute 6 record your pulse rate and the loading wattage
- Use the Astrand-Ryhming Nomogram to determine your VO2
- Multiply your VO2 value by 1000 and divide by your weight (kg) to determine your VO2 max
- The calculator below will provide you with an estimate of your VO2 max L and VO2 max ksg/ml/min

Analysis

Analysis of the result is by comparing it with the results of previous tests. It is expected that, with appropriate training between each test, the analysis would indicate an improvement.

106

Multi-Stage Fitness Test

Objective

The objective of the Multi-Stage Fitness Test (MSFT) is to monitor the development of the athlete's maximum oxygen uptake (VO2 max).

This test is very good for games players as it is specific to the nature of the sport but, due to the short turns, is perhaps not suitable for rowers, runners or cyclists.

Required Resources

To undertake this test you will require :

A flat, non slippery surface at least 20 metres in length

30 metre tape measure

Marking cones

Pre-recorded audio tape or CD

Tape recorder or CD Player

Recording sheets

Assistant

The Multi-Stage Fitness Test audio tape or CD can be purchased from Coachwise 1st4Sport.

How to conduct the test

The test is made up of 23 levels where each level lasts approx. one minute. Each level comprises of a series of 20m shuttles where the starting speed is 8.5km/hr and increases by 0.5km/hr at each level. On the tape a single beep indicates the end of a shuttle and 3 beeps indicates the start of the next level. The test is conducted as follows:

- Measure out a 20 metres section and mark each end with a marker cone
- The athlete carries out a warm up program of jogging and stretching exercises
- The test is conducted
    - The athlete must place one foot on or beyond the 20m marker at the end of each shuttle
    - If the athlete arrives at the end of a shuttle before the beep, the athlete must wait for the beep and then resume running
    - The athlete keeps running for as long as possible until he/she can longer keep up with the speed set by the tape at which point they should voluntarily withdraw.
    - If the athlete fails to reach the end of the shuttle before the beep they should be allowed 2 or 3 further shuttles to attempt to regain the required pace before being withdrawn
    - Record the level and number of shuttles completed at that level by the athlete
    - At the end of the test the athletes conduct a cool down program, including stretching exercises

Analysis

Analysis of the result is by comparing it with the results of previous tests. It is expected that, with appropriate training between each test, the analysis would indicate an improvement.

Performance Assessment

The athlete's maximum oxygen uptake (VO2 max) can be determined from the MSF Table using the Level and Shuttle achieved.

The calculator below will provide you with an estimate of your VO2 max. Please note that, when compared to the MSF Table values, the calculator result can be in error by up to ± 0.3 mls/kg/min.

Normative data for MSFT

Table 31 national team scores for the MSFT

Sport	*Male*	*Female*
Basketball	L11 - S5	L9 - S6
Hockey	L13 - S9	L12 - S7
Rugby League	L13 - S1	
Netball		L9 - S7
Squash	L13 - S13	

Table Reference: Beashel P. et al; The world of sport examined; 1997.

Notes

A degree of caution is required in administering the test, in that you have to push yourself relatively hard to the point where you can no longer maintain the pace dictated by the tape. If you are suffering from any injury or illness, or if you have any reason to think you may not be in a good general state of health, you should consult a doctor before doing this test.

As the audio-tapes may stretch over time, the tapes need to be calibrated which involves timing a one-minute interval and making adjustment to the distance between markers. The recording is also available on compact disc, which does not require calibration.

Knowing that the starting speed is 8.5km/hr and increases by 0.5km/hr at each level then the time for each 20 metre section, at each level, can be estimated from the following equation:

- 20m Time = 72 ÷ (((Level - 1) × 0.5) + 8.5)

The time for 20m at level 11 is 5.33 seconds.

Knowing that the starting speed is 8.5km/hr and increases by 0.5km/hr at each level and the duration of each level is approximately one minute then the number of shuttles at each level, can be estimated from the following equation:

- Shuttles = (((Level - 1) × 0.5) + 8.5) × 0.838

The result is rounded up to the nearest whole number e.g. the number of shuttles at level 17 is 13.82 which is rounded up to 14 shuttles.

107

Body Fat From Girth

Measuring body fat percentage is an easy method of discovering correct body weight and composition. Beneath the skin is a layer of subcutaneous fat, and the percentage of total body fat can be measured by taking the girth measurements at selected points on the body with a measuring tape.

Measurement Sites

Depending on your age and gender three body measurements (sites) can be used for determining your percentage body fat.

Table 32

Age (years)	*Gender*	*Site A*	*Site B*	*Site C*
18 - 26	Male	Right Upper Arm	Abdomen	Right Forearm
	Female	Abdomen	Right Thigh	Right Forearm
27 - 50	Male	Buttocks	Abdomen	Right Forearm
	Female	Abdomen	Right Thigh	Right Calf

The measurement sites are as follows:

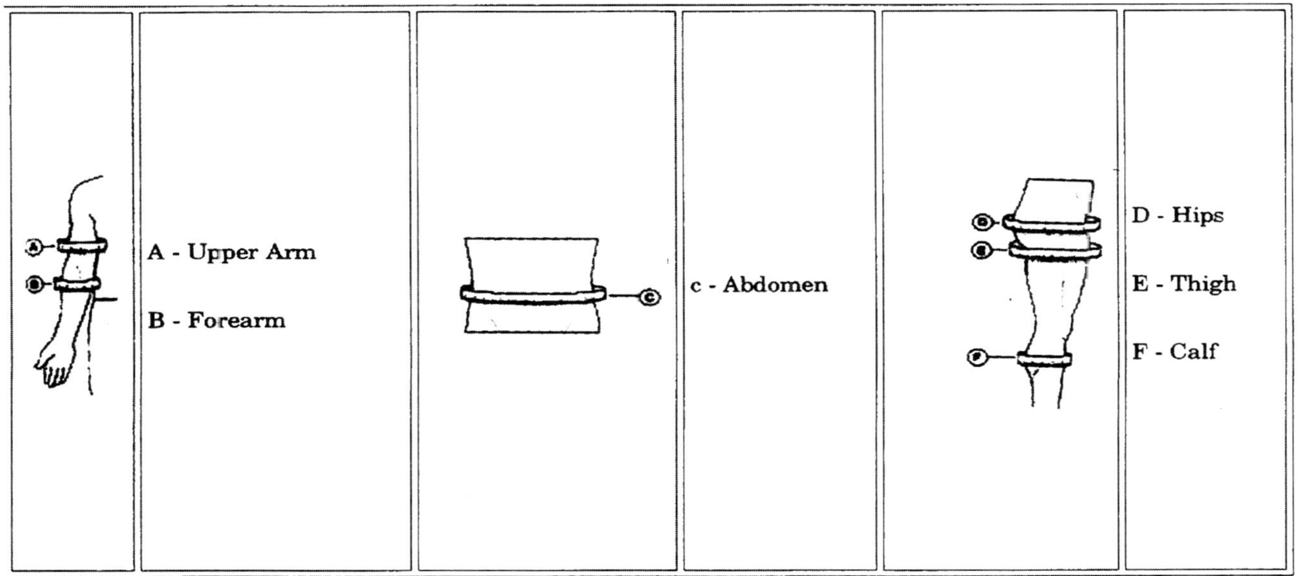

Fig. 42 - Body Fat

Method

The method is as follows:

Based on your age range and gender determine the required three measurement sites from the table above

Record the measurements in centimetres of these three sites (A, B, C)

Use the calculator below to determine your percentage body fat

Typical Scores

The average man has 15 to 17% body fat, while the average woman is between 18 and 22%. Typical scores for elite athletes are 6% to 12% for men and 12% to 20% for women.

The following table details the percentage body fat for male and female athletes for a variety of sports.

Table 33 : Body Fat

Sport	*Male*	*Female*
Baseball	12-15%	12-18%
Basketball	6-12%	20-27%
Canoe/Kayak	6-12%	10-16%
Cycling	5-15%	15-20%
Field & Ice Hockey	8-15%	12-18%
Gymnastics	5-12%	10-16%
Rowing	6-14%	12-18%
Swimming	9-12%	14-24%
Tennis	12-16%	16-24%
Track - Runners	8-10%	12-20%
Track - Jumpers	7-12%	10-18%
Track - Throwers	14-20%	20-28%
Triathlon	5-12%	10-15%
Volleyball	11-14%	16-25%

Your Ideal Weight

The most accurate assessment of your ideal weight takes into account the composition of your body - how much of your weight is lean body mass (muscle and bone) and how much is body fat. For optimum health, body fat should be no more than 20% of total body weight for men and 30% for women.

Ideal Weight Table

The following table is a guide to a healthy weight range for each height and sex group. The table does not take into consideration your age or your frame size. A person with a petite physique ought to aim for an ideal weight at the lower end of the range. A person of the same height but with a larger frame could quite satisfactorily weigh in at the top of the range.

Table 34 : Ideal Weight

Height		*Men*		*Women*	
Feet & Inches	*Metres*	*Kg*	*lbs*	*Kg*	*lbs*
4' 7"	1.40	...	...	40 - 53	88 - 116
4' 9"	1.45	...	...	42 - 54	92 - 119
4' 11"	1.50	...	...	43 - 55	94 - 121
4' 11½"	1.52	...	...	44 - 56	97 - 123
5' ½"	1.54	...	...	44 - 57	97 - 125
5' 1"	1.56	...	...	45 - 58	99 - 128
5' 2"	1.58	51 - 64	112 - 141	46 - 59	101 - 130
5' 2½"	1.60	52 - 65	114 - 143	48 - 61	105 - 134
5' 3½"	1.62	53 - 66	116 - 145	49 - 62	108 - 136
5' 4½"	1.64	54 - 67	119 - 147	50 - 64	110 - 141
5' 5"	1.66	55 - 69	121 - 152	51 - 65	112 - 143
5' 6"	1.68	56 - 71	123 - 156	52 - 66	114 - 145
5' 6½"	1.70	58 - 73	127 - 161	53 - 67	117 - 147
5' 7½"	1.72	59 - 74	130 - 163	55 - 69	121 - 152
5' 8½"	1.74	60 - 75	132 - 165	56 - 70	123 - 154
5' 9"	1.76	62 - 77	136 - 169	58 - 72	128 - 158
5' 10"	1.78	64 - 79	141 - 174	59 - 74	130 - 163
5' 11½"	1.80	65 - 80	143 - 176	...	...

(Contd.)

(Contd. Table 34)

Height		*Men*		*Women*	
6' 0"	1.84	67 - 84	147 - 185	...	...
6' 1"	1.86	69 - 86	152 - 189	...	...
6' 2"	1.88	71 - 88	156 - 194	...	...
6' 2½"	1.90	73 - 90	161 - 198	...	...
6' 3½"	1.92	75 - 93	165 - 205	...	...

108

Bruce Treadmill Test

Objective

To monitor the development of the athlete's general endurance (VO2 max).

Required Resources

To undertake this test you will require:

Treadmill where speed and grade of slope can be adjusted

Stop watch

Assistant

Analysis

Analysis of the result is by comparing it with the results of previous tests. It is expected that, with appropriate training between each test, the analysis would indicate an improvement

How to conduct the test

The athlete runs on a treadmill to exhaustion. At timed stages during the test the speed (km/hr) and grade of slope (%) of the treadmill are increased as detailed in the table below.

Active and sedentary men - Foster et al. 1984

From the total walk/run time an estimate of the athlete's VO2 max can be calculated as follows:

$$VO2\ max = 14.8 - (1.379 \times T) + (0.451 \times T^2) - (0.012 \times T^3)$$

Table 35 : Treadmill Ressistance

Stage	Time (min)	km/hr	Slope
1	0	2.74	10%
2	3	4.02	12%
3	6	5.47	14%
4	9	6.76	16%
5	12	8.05	18%
6	15	8.85	20%
7	18	9.65	22%
8	21	10.46	24%
9	24	11.26	26%
10	27	12.07	28%

The treadmill is set up with the Stage 1 speed (2.74 km/hr) and grade of slope (10%) and the athlete commences the test.

At the appropriate times during the test, the speed and slope of the treadmill are adjusted.

Therefore after 3 minutes into the test the speed is adjusted to 4.02 km/hr and the slope to 12%, after 6 minutes into the test the speed is adjusted to 5.47 km/hr and the slope to 14%, and so on.

The assistant starts the stopwatch at the start of the test and stops it when the athlete is unable to continue - this ideally should be between 9 and 15 minutes.

"T" is the total time of the test expressed in minutes and fractions of a minute e.g. 13 minutes 15 seconds=13.25 minutes

109

Burpee Test

Objective

The objective of this test is to monitor the development of the athlete's agility and balance.

Required Resources

To undertake this test you will require:

- Non slip surface
- Stop watch
- An assistant

How to conduct the test

The athlete practices the technique which involves:
standing erect, arms by the side
placing the hands on the floor in front of the feet (squat position)
thrusting the legs back to assume a push up position with a straight line from the shoulders to the heels
returning to the squat position
returning to the starting position
The athlete performs as many repetitions as possible in 15 seconds
A point is given for every successfully completed repetition
Half a point is deducted for each repetition in which poor technique is demonstrated, such as: not resuming the erect position. kicking

the feet back prior to hand placement not assuming a straight push up body position

Analysis

Analysis of the result is by comparing it with the results of previous tests. It is expected that, with appropriate training between each test, the analysis would indicate an improvement.

110

Fat-free Body Mass and Lean Body Mass

The fat-free body mass (FFBM) represents the body mass devoid of all fat whereas lean body mass (LBM) contains a small percentage of essential fat. LBM is a theoretical value developed by Behnke. For men Behnke considered it to be FFBM+3% essential fat and for females FFBM+12% fat (3% essential fat + 9% sex specific essential fat). Many researches use the terms FFBM and LBM interchangeably.

Typical Scores

The average male has 15 to 17% body fat, while the average female is between 18 and 22%. Typical scores for elite athletes are 6% to 12% for men and 12% to 20% for women.

The following table details the percentage body fat for male and female athletes for a variety of sports.

Table 36 : Fat Free Body Mass

Sport	*Male*	*Female*
Baseball	12-15%	12-18%
Basketball	6-12%	20-27%
Cycling	5-15%	15-20%
Field & Ice Hockey	8-15%	12-18%
Rowing	6-14%	12-18%
Swimming	9-12%	14-24%
Track - Runners	8-10%	12-20%
Track - Jumpers	7-12%	10-18%
Track - Throwers	14-20%	20-28%
Triathlon	5-12%	10-15%
Volleyball	11-14%	16-15%

111

Competitive Anxiety

Competition can cause athletes to react both physically (somatic) and mentally (cognitive) in a manner which can negatively affect their performance abilities. Stress, arousal and anxiety are terms used to describe this condition.

How do you measure it?

A range of psychometric tests or sport anxiety questionnaires (SAQ) have been used by sports psychologists to understand and measure this condition. In 1966 Charles Spielberger argued that it was necessary to make a distinction between momentary states and more permanent traits.

Anxiety states (A-state) is our response to a particular situation (i.e. sky diving).

Anxiety traits (A-trait) are the characteristics of our personality, our general anxiety level

Marten developed anxiety traits (A-trait) questionnaires that were tailored specially to sport known as the Sport Competition Anxiety Test (SCAT). Marten recognised that any measure of sport anxiety must take into consideration cognitive anxiety (negative thoughts, worry) and somatic anxiety (physiological response).

The Competitive State Anxiety Inventory or CSAI-2 takes into account the difference between A-state and A-trait and distinguishes between cognitive and somatic anxiety.

Controlling Anxiety

As we can see anxiety includes state and trait dimensions both of which can show themselves as cognitive and somatic symptoms. An athlete with high anxiety trait (A-trait) is likely to be more anxious in stressful situations. To help the athlete control competitive anxiety somatic techniques (relaxation) and cognitive techniques (mental imagery) can be used.

Anxiety - Performance relationship

Drive Theory

According to the Drive Theory (Clark Hull 1943) if an athlete is appropriately skilled then it will help them to perform well if their drive to compete is aroused - they are "psyched up".

Inverted-U hypothesis

An alternative approach to Drive Theory is known as the Inverted-U hypothesis that predicts a relationship between arousal and performance approximates to an inverted U shape. The theory is that as arousal is increased then performance improves but only up to a certain point (top of the inverted U). If the athlete's arousal is increased beyond this point then performance diminishes.

Multi-dimensional Anxiety Theory

Multi-dimensional Anxiety Theory is based on the distinction between cognitive anxiety and somatic anxiety. The theory makes a series of predictions:

There will be a negative but linear relationship between cognitive anxiety and performance

There will be an inverted U relationship between somatic anxiety and performance

Somatic anxiety should decline once performance begins but cognitive anxiety may remain high if confidence is low

Catastrophe Theory

Catastrophe Theory suggests that:

Stress and anxiety will influence performance each athlete will respond in a unique way to competitive anxiety performance will be effected in a unique way which may be difficult to predict using general rules

Optimum Arousal Theory

According to the Optimum Arousal Theory (Yuri Hanin) each athlete will perform at their best if their level of arousal or competitive anxiety falls within their optimum functioning zone. The challenge for the coach is to determine the athlete's zone and identify the techniques that will place the athlete in this zone prior to competition.

112

Conconi Test

Objective

The Conconi test (Conconi et al, 1982) is a simple method for measuring the approximate values of an individual's maximum, anaerobic and aerobic threshold rates. This test has been shown to be flawed (Jones and Doust, 1995).

Required Resources

To perform the test you require

A Heart Rate Monitor (HRM)

A 400 metre track or Treadmill

Stop watch

Assistant to record 200 metre times and heart rate

Before you start the test you need to determine your starting speed and how much you increment your speed by every 200 metres.

Using your best 10 km time the Conconi Test Pace Calculator can determine the time for each 200 metres for the track test and the speed for the treadmill test.

Conducting the Conconi Test on a 400m Track

In the Conconi test, the athlete increases their speed gradually every 200 metres and the heart rate and time, at each

200 metre point, are recorded. This gradual increase in speed every 200 metres is maintained until the athlete is unable to maintain the pace. The total distance covered by the test should be between 2.5 km and 4 km to ensure sufficient information is available for subsequent calculations. Speed versus heart rate is then plotted on a graph from which the athlete's anaerobic threshold can be determined.

- Perform a five to ten minute warm up program
- Set the HRM to use a 5 second recording interval
- Start the HRM watch at the starting point
- Every 200 metres record the time and heart rate
- Every 200 metres increase your speed
- End the test when you can no longer maintain the pace
- Stop the HRM recording
- Perform a 10 minute cool down program

Conducting the Conconi Test on a Treadmill

- Perform a five to ten minute warm up program
- Set the HRM to use a 5 second recording interval
- Start the treadmill speed at the required start speed
- Start the HRM stop watch
- Record the time and heart rate every 200 metres
- Increase the treadmill speed every 200 metres by 0.5km/hr
- End the test when you have reached your maximum heart rate or you can continue no longer
- Stop the HRM recording
- Perform a 10 minute cool down program

Calculation of Anaerobic Threshold

Determine the speed for each 200 metres and then for each 200 metres plot speed versus heart rate on a graph. You will find the graph gradually rises to start with and then flattens before rising again. This flattening in the graph indicates the athlete's anaerobic threshold. In the example conconi graph below this flattening appears to be around 182 bpm.

Alternatively you can use the supplied Conconi AT Calculator to plot and determine the athlete's Anaerobic Threshold.

Table 37 : Conconi Test

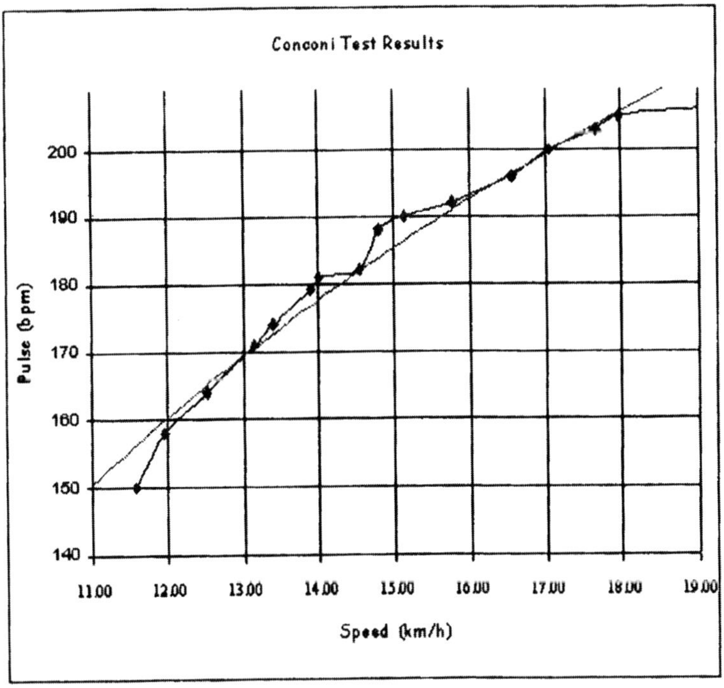

113

Core Muscle Strength and Stability Test

Objective

The objective of the Core Muscle Strength and Stability Test is to monitor the development of the athlete's abdominal and lower back muscles.

Required Resources

To undertake this test you will require :

- Flat surface
- Mat
- Watch

How to conduct the test

The Core Muscle Strength and Stability Test is conducted as follows:

- Position the watch on the ground where you can easily see it
- Assume the basic press up position (elbows on the ground) - as in the picture above
- Hold this position for 60 seconds

Fig. 43 : Core Muscle Strength

- Lift your right arm off the ground
- Hold this position for 15 seconds
- Return your right arm to the ground and lift the left arm off the ground
- Hold this position for 15 seconds
- Return your left arm to the ground and lift the right leg off the ground
- Hold this position for 15 seconds
- Return your right leg to the ground and lift the left leg off the ground
- Hold this position for 15 seconds
- Lift your left leg and right arm off the ground
- Hold this position for 15 seconds
- Return you left leg and right arm to the ground
- Lift your right leg and left arm off the ground
- Hold this position for 15 seconds
- Return to the basic press up position (elbows on the ground) - as in the picture above
- Hold this position for 30 seconds

114

Curl-up Test

Objective

The objective of the Curl-Up Test is to assess the endurance of the athlete's abdominal muscles.

Required Resources

To undertake this test you will require:

- flat surface
- mat
- watch
- a partner

How to conduct the test

The Sit Ups Test is conducted as follows:

Lie on the mat with the knees bent, feet flat on the floor, the hands resting on the thighs and the back of the head on the partner's hands- see Figure 1

Curl up slowly using the abdominal muscles and slide the hands up the thighs until the finger tips touch the knee caps - see Figure 2

Return slowly to the starting position - see Figure 1

The feet are not to be held

A complete curl-up is to take 3 seconds - that is 20 repetitions/ minute

Repeat as many curls as possible at this rate

Record the total number of curls

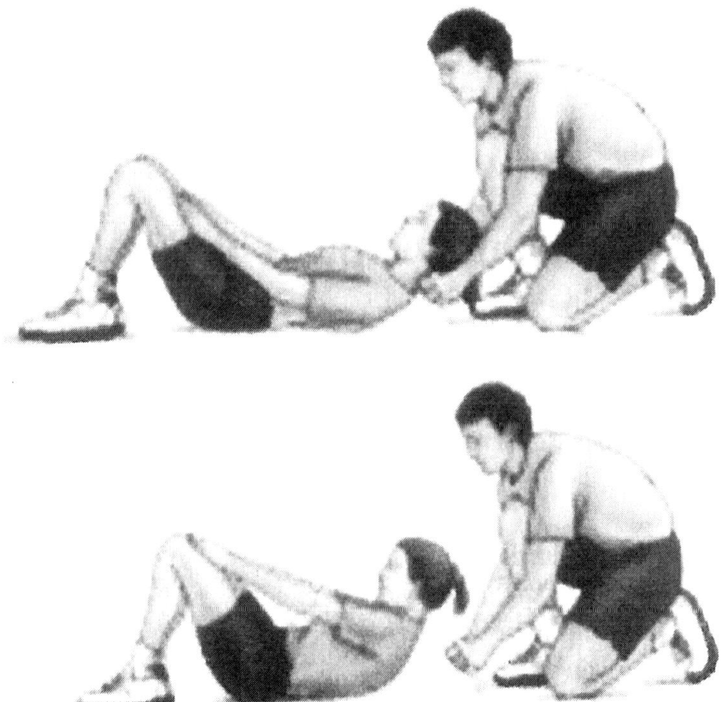

Fig. 44 : Curl Up

Analysis

Analysis of the result is by comparing it with the results of previous tests. It is expected that, with appropriate training between each test, the analysis would indicate an improvement.

115

400m Drop Off Test

Objective

The objective of this test is to monitor the athlete's anaerobic efficiency.

Required Resources

To undertake this test you will require:

400m track

Stop watch

An assistant

How to conduct the test

The test is conducted as follows:

The athlete is timed running at full speed over 100 metres

The athlete takes a five-minute recovery

The athlete is timed running at full speed over 400m

The time for the 400m is converted to 100m splits by dividing the time by 4

The 100 metre sprint time is then subtracted from the split-time, giving the drop off time

Analysis

Analysis of the result is by comparing it with the results of previous tests. It is expected that, with appropriate training between each test, the analysis would indicate an improvement.

Example

100m time = 13.0 seconds

400m time = 60.0 seconds

60 ÷ 4 = 15 seconds

15 - 13 = a drop off time of 2 seconds

The aim is always to reduce the 'drop off' time by increasing anaerobic efficiency. A top female 400m runner has a 'drop off' time of around 0.7 seconds.

116

Leg Strength Test - Dynamic

Objective

To monitor the development of the athlete's elastic leg strength.

Required Resources

To undertake this test you will require:

400 metre track - 25 metre marked section on the straight
Cones
Stop Watch
Assistant

How to conduct the test

Mark out a 25 metre section on the straight section of the track with two cones. The athlete starts 10 to 15 metres behind the starting line. Using a jog run up, the athlete starts hopping on the dominant leg from the first cone. The time taken to hop between the two cones is recorded. The test is then repeated with the other leg.

Analysis

Analysis of the result is by comparing it with the results of previous tests. It is expected that, with appropriate training between each test, the analysis would indicate an improvement.

Normative data for the Leg Strength Test

The following data has been obtained from the results of tests conducted with world class athletes.

Table 38 : Leg Stength Score

% Rank	*Females*	*Males*
91-100	3.13 - 3.75 secs	2.70 - 3.25 secs
81 - 90	3.76 - 4.50 secs	3.36 - 3.90 secs
71 - 80	4.51 - 5.70 secs	3.91 - 5.00 secs
61 - 70	5.71 - 6.90 secs	5.01 - 6.10 secs
51 - 60	6.91 - 8.15 secs	6.11 - 7.20 secs
41 - 50	8.16 - 8.90 secs	7.21 - 7.90 secs
31 - 40	8.91 - 9.45 secs	7.91 - 8.40 secs
21 - 30	9.46 - 10.05 secs	8.41 - 8.95 secs
11 - 20	10.06 - 10.34 secs	8.96 - 9.25 secs
1 - 10	10.35 - 10.70 secs	9.26 - 9.60 secs

117

Yuhasz Skinfold Test

Measuring body fat percentage is an easy method of discovering correct body weight and composition. Beneath the skin is a layer of subcutaneous fat, and the percentage of total body fat can be measured by taking the 'skinfold' at selected points on the body with a pair of callipers. The Yuhasz Technique uses six sites as opposed to the three of four sites used in many other tests.

Method

The method is as follows:

Ensure that all of the skinfold measurements are located on the right side of the body and that the measurements are taken in millimetres.

Pick up the skinfold between the thumb and the index finger so as to include two thicknesses of skin and subcutaneous fat.

Apply the callipers about one centimetre from the fingers and at a depth about equal to the thickness of the fold.

Very slightly release the pressure of the fingers so the greater pressure is exerted by the caliper.

Repeat the procedure three times as the measurement may vary and take an average.

In order to standardise, measurements should be taken by the same person and at the same time of day, preferably in the morning.

Add the results of each measurement to get a total value in millimetres.

Using the calculator below to determine the percentage body fat.

Measurement Sites

The following sites are used for determining percentage body fat:

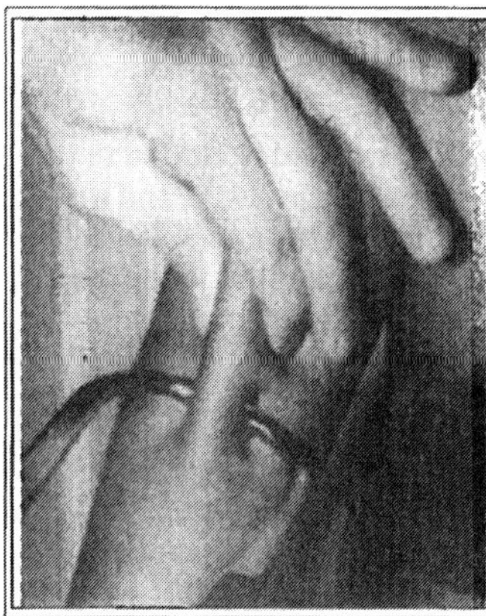

Triceps

The skin fold is located midway on the back of the upper arm. The arm hangs freely and the skinfold is lifted parallel to its long axis.

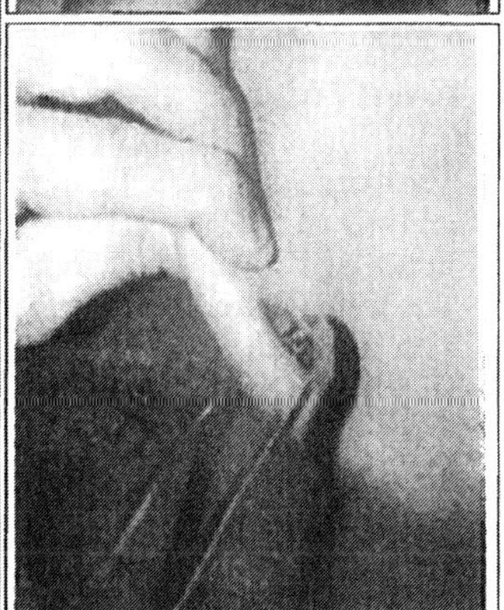

Subscapula

The skinfold is lifted vertically and measured below the tip of the scapula.

Fig. 45 : Skinfold

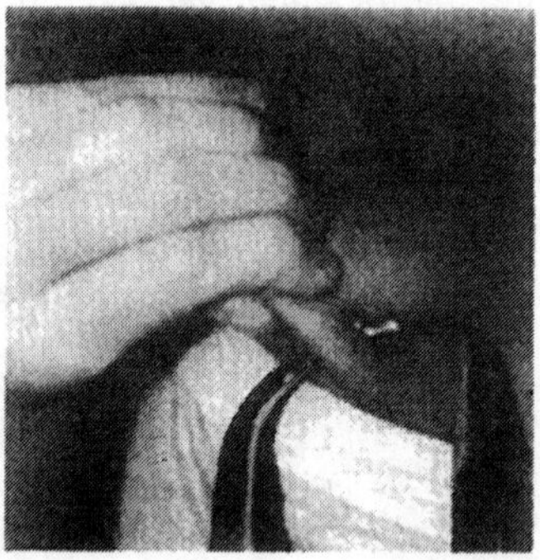

Suprailiac

The skinfold is located immediately above the crest of the ilium. The fold is lifted at a slight angle to the vertical along the normal fold line.

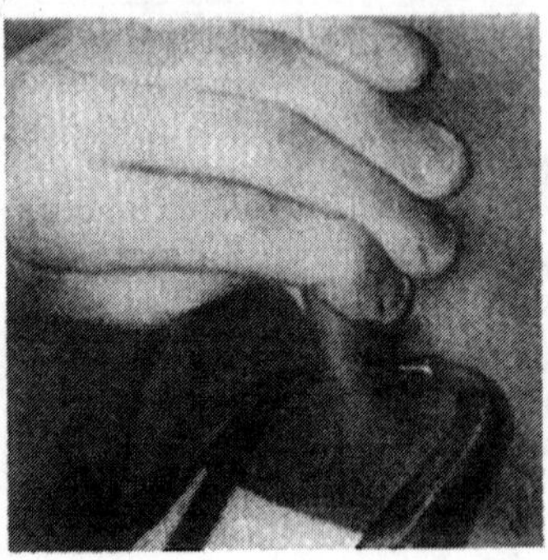

Abdomen

The skinfold is located to the left of, adjacent to, and in line with the navel. The fold is lifted parallel to the long axis of the body.

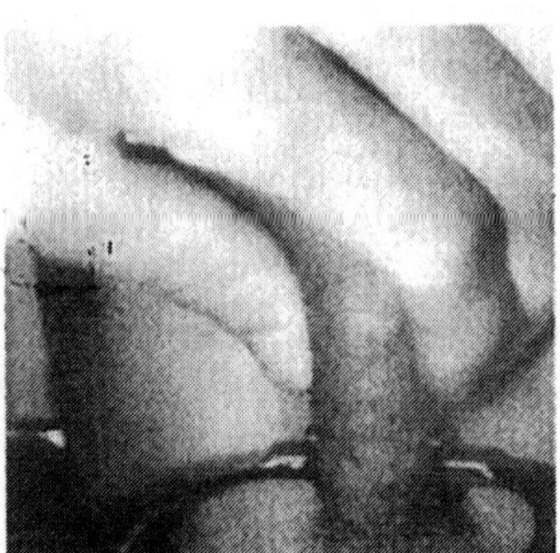

Front Thigh

The skinfold is located midway on the front of the upper leg over the quadriceps. The foot is placed on a six-inch step with the knee slightly flexed and muscles relaxed. The fold is lifted parallel to the long axis of the leg.

Fig. 46 : Skinfold

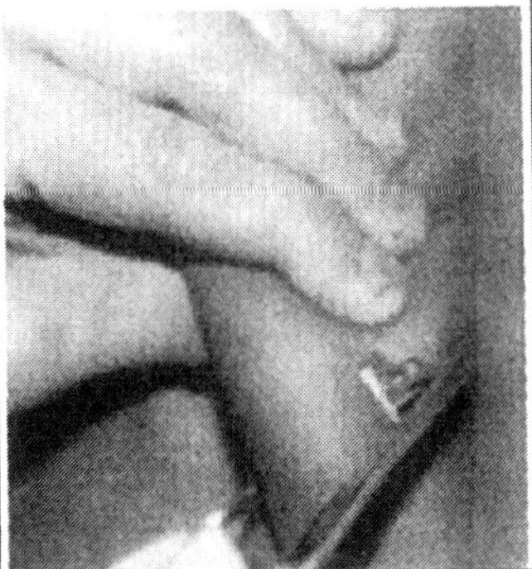

Chest (male only)

The site is located above and slightly to the right of the right nipple. The skinfold is taken at a 45-degree angle of the horizontal.

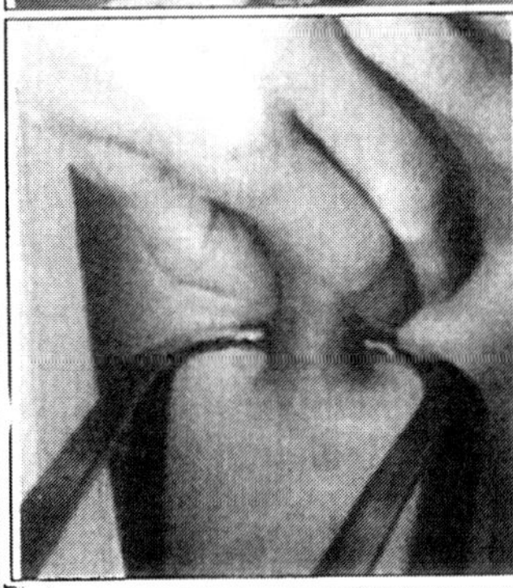

Rear thigh (female only)

The skinfold is located midway on the back of the upper leg. The leg is held in the same position as the front thigh measurements. The skinfold is lifted parallel to the axis of the leg.

Fig. 47 : Skinfold

118

250 Metre Endurance Test

Objective

To monitor the development of the athlete's endurance for the 200 metres event.

Required Resources

To undertake this test you will require:

400 metre track - 250 metre marked section

Stop watch

Assistant

How to conduct the test

The test comprises of a 250 metre run from a standing start. The assistant records the time for the athlete to complete 250 metres.

Analysis

Analysis of the result is by comparing it with the results of previous tests. It is expected that, with appropriate training between each test, the analysis would indicate an improvement.

119

1500 Metre Predictor Test

Objective

The 1500 metre Predictor Test is used to predict an athlete's 1500 metre time.

Required Resources

To undertake this test you will require:

400 metre track

Stop watch

An assistant

How to conduct the test

The athlete is required to run 2 sets of

400 metres

45 seconds Recovery

800 metres

90 seconds Recovery

300 metres

3 minutes Recovery

The time for each run is recorded and the accumulated time for each set is recorded. The average time of these two accumulated times is the predicted 1500 metres time for the athlete.

Example

Set 1

400 metres in 63 seconds

800 metres in 129 seconds

300 metres in 48 seconds

Accumulated time for set 1 is 240 seconds (4 minutes)

Set 2

400 metres in 67 seconds

800 metres in 164 seconds

300 metres in 52 seconds

Accumulated time for set 2 is 283 seconds (4 minutes 43 seconds)

Average time of the two accumulated times is (240 + 283) ÷ 2 = 261.5 seconds

Predicted time for the 1500 metres is 4 minutes 21.5 seconds

When to use

To predict performance and monitor progress this test can be used at the:

beginning of the winter training to establish a baseline (September/October)

just prior to indoor racing (December/January)

just prior to the outdoor season (March/April)

Analysis

Analysis of the result is by comparing it with the results of previous tests. It is expected that, with appropriate training between each test, the analysis would indicate an improvement.

120

40 Metre Multiple Sprint Test

Objective

The objective of this test is to monitor the athlete's level of sprint fatigue.

Required Resources

To undertake this test you will require:

400 metre track - with a 40 metre marked section on the straight
Starting Blocks
Stop watch
An assistant

How to conduct the test

The test comprises of 6 × 40 metre runs from a standing start or from starting blocks and with a 30 second recovery between each run. The assistant should record the time for the athlete to complete the 40 metres.

Analysis

The quickest sprint time is multiplied by 6 to give an optimal sprint time. The difference between the total and optimal times indicates the level of fatigue experienced in the performer.

Analysis of the result is by comparing it with the results of previous tests. It is expected that, with appropriate training between each test, the analysis would indicate an improvement.

121

400 Metre Control Tests

Objective

To monitor the speed, speed endurance, strength/general endurance of a 400 metre athlete.

Required Resources

To undertake this test you will require:

- 400 metre track
- Cones to mark 150 metre, 300 metre and 600 metre points
- Stop watch
- Assistant

How to conduct the test

The test comprises of three separate runs over 150 metres, 300 metres and 600 metres from a standing start and with a full recovery between each run. The assistant should record the time for the athlete to complete each distance.

Analysis

Analysis of the result is by comparing it with the results of previous tests. It is expected that, with appropriate training between each test, the analysis would indicate an improvement.

Speed Endurance Index

If the athlete's speed endurance index is greater than the target index value, and provided the 150 metre time is in line with training targets, then more speed endurance work (lactic anaerobic) is indicated.

Strength and General Endurance Index

If the athlete's strength and general endurance index is greater than the target index value, and provided the 300 metre time is in line with training targets, then more strength and general endurance work (aerobic) is indicated.

122

400m Predictor Test

Objective

Frank Horwill's 40 yard (36. 6 metres) test is used to predict an athlete's potential 400 metre

Required Resources

To undertake this test you will require:

- 400 metre track
- Stop watch
- An assistant

How to conduct the test

- The athlete is required to run 40 yards (36.6 metres) from a crouch start
- The assistance records the time
- Repeat the test 2 or 3 times and note the best time

  The athlete's potential 400m time, in seconds, can be calculated as follows:
- Male athletes = (Time for 40 yards × 10) + 2
- Female athletes = (Time for 40 yards × 10) + 4

123

5 km Predictor Test

Objective

The 5km Predictor Test is used to predict an athlete's 5 kilometre time.

Required Resources

To undertake this test you will require:

- 400 metre track
- Stop watch
- An assistant

How to conduct the test

The athlete is required to run 4 × 1600 metres with 90 seconds recovery between each run and the time for each 1600 metres is recorded.

Calculate the average of the 4 recorded times and multiply the result by 3.125. The result is the predicted 5km time for the athlete.

The 3.125 comes from the fact the average time is for 1600 metres and we require a time for 5000 metres hence we need to divide the time by 1600 and multiply the result by 5000 (5000 ÷ 1600=3.125)

Example

The recorded times for each 1600 metres are:

- 4 minutes 5 seconds
- 4 minutes 10 seconds
- 4 minutes 18 seconds
- 4 minutes 32 seconds

Average time of the four runs is 4 minutes 16.25 seconds (256.25 seconds)

Multiply the result by 3.125 = 13 minutes 20.8 seconds

Predicted time for the 5km is 13 minutes 20.8 seconds

124

505 Agility Test

Objective

The objective of this test is to monitor the development of the athlete's speed and agility.

Required Resources

To undertake this test you will require:

6 cones
Non slip surface
Stopwatch
An assistant

How to conduct the test

- Mark out the course as per the diagram above. The distance from A to B is 10 metres and the distance from B to C is 5 metres.
- The athlete runs from the start line (A) towards the 10 metre line (B) (run in distance to build up speed).
- The assistant starts the stopwatch as the athlete passes through the 10 metre line (B).
- The athlete runs on to the 15 metre line (C), turns and runs back towards the start line.

- The assistant stops the stopwatch when the athlete passes through the 10 metre line (B) on their return to the start line.
- The best of two trails is recorded.

125

Quick Feet Test

Objective

The quick feet test provides information on the presence of fast-twitch muscle fibre in the muscles involved in sprinting and indicates your potential to execute quick movements. Hereditary factors such as limb length, muscle attachments, and proportion of fast-twitch fibres do place a limit on one's maximum potential, but we can improve our speed and quickness with proper training.

Normative Data

Speed through a ladder can indicate much about an athlete's quickness. A time of less than 2.8 seconds for males and 3.4 seconds for females for running the length of a 20 rung ladder, one foot in each rung at a time, is considered as excellent for college athletes.

Table 39 : Quick Feet Test - Male

Males	*Time*
Jnr High School	< 3.8 seconds
Snr High School	< 3.3 seconds
College	< 2.8 seconds

Table 40 : Quick Feet Test - Female

Females	*Time*
Jnr High School	< 4.2 seconds
Snr High School	< 3.8 seconds
College	< 3.4 seconds

126

Flexed Arm-Hang Test

Testing and measurement are the means of collecting information upon which subsequent performance evaluations and decisions are made but in the analysis we need to bear in mind the factors that may influence the results.

Objective

The objective of this test is to monitor the muscular endurance of the athlete's elbow flexors and shoulder extensors.

Required Resources

To undertake this test you will require:

- Bar above head height
- Stopwatch
- Assistant

How to conduct the test

- Athlete uses a flexed arm hang position using a supinated grip (palm facing the subject) grip. The chin is above the bar, hips and knees are extended
- Once the athlete is in position the assistant start the stopwatch
- The athlete attempts to maintain this position for as long as possible (maximum time is 30 seconds)

- The timing is stopped when the chin drops below the top of the bar or 30 seconds elapse
- The assistant records number of seconds that the flexed arm-hang position can be maintained (maximum of 30 seconds).

Analysis

Analysis of the result is by comparing it with the results of previous tests. It is expected that, with appropriate training between each test, the analysis would indicate an improvement.

127

Flying 30 metre Test

Testing and measurement are the means of collecting information upon which subsequent performance evaluations and decisions are made but in the analysis we need to bear in mind the factors that may influence the results.

Objective

To monitor the development of the athlete's maximum speed.

Required Resources

To undertake this test you will require:
400 metre track - 60 metre marked section on the straight
Cone to mark 30m point
Stop watch
Assistant

How to conduct the test

The test comprises of 3 × 60 metre runs from a standing start and with a full recovery between each run. The athlete uses the first 30 metres to build up to maximum speed and then maintains the speed through to 60 metres. This test can be combined with the 60 metre speed test. The assistant records the time for the athlete to complete the:

- first 30 metres
- whole 60 metres

Analysis

Analysis of the result is by comparing it with the results of previous tests. It is expected that, with appropriate training between each test, the analysis would indicate an improvement.

Normative data for the Flying 30 metre test

The following data has been obtained from the results of tests conducted with world class athletes.

Table 41 : Flying 30 Metre Test

% Rank	*Females*	*Males*
91-100	2.90 - 2.99 seconds	2.50 - 2.59 seconds
81 - 90	3.00 - 3.09 seconds	2.60 - 2.69 seconds
71 - 80	3.10 - 3.19 seconds	2.70 - 2.79 seconds
61 - 70	3.20 - 3.29 seconds	2.80 - 2.89 seconds
51 - 60	3.30 - 3.39 seconds	2.90 - 2.99 seconds
41 - 50	3.40 - 3.49 seconds	3.00 - 3.09 seconds
31 - 40	3.50 - 3.59 seconds	3.10 - 3.19 seconds
21 - 30	3.60 - 3.69 seconds	3.20 - 3.29 seconds
11 - 20	3.70 - 3.79 seconds	3.30 -3.39 seconds
1 - 10	3.80 - 3.89 seconds	3.40 - 3.49 seconds

Table reference: D.A. Chu; Explosive Power and Strength; Human Kinetics; 1996.

Maximum Heart Rate Stress Tests

Many athletes who have a history of continual sport since their early teens have a higher maximum heart rate when compared to the mathematical calculation of their maximum heart rate based on their age. To be certain of finding your maximum heart rate a Stress Test should be conducted.

128

Maximum Heart Rate Stress Tests

Anyone who has undergone a stress test will know that it is not easy. A stress test although relatively short does require you to push your body and your heart to the very limit. Before undertaking a stress test, you should be certain of the following:

- that you have not suffered from any cold, flu, stomach bug or other illness in the last six to eight weeks. The body in this period could still be fighting the last of the infection and the effort of a stress test could leave you prone to a more serious infection. If in any doubt check with your doctor
- that you have not raced in the fourteen days prior to a stress test and at least four to six weeks following a marathon or more if you have not yet fully recovered from your efforts. A tired heart and body will not achieve maximum
- in the final week before a stress test it is important to recovery run - that is 70% maximum of your current age adjusted heart rate
- Do not undertake a stress test:
- with any hint of an injury. Ensure all old injuries are fully repaired before deciding to undertake stress test
- if you have less than one years running experience and are sport active for less than three hours a week. It is possible

you will not be fit enough to take the strain of a stress test let alone achieve a reliable result.

Any one who is overweight or over the age of 35 is advised to see their doctor before under going a stress test. I hope that you get the idea that a maximum heart rate stress test is not easy. It is the very limit of your heart and bodies capability and should not be treated lightly.

The tests will require you to wear your heart rate monitor (HRM) and preferable one that is capable of recording your heart rate. It is best to record your heart rate as often as possible - preferable every second or at worst every 5 seconds. If your HRM does not have a record facility, it will be necessary to keep glancing at your monitor to find your highest heart rate. For both these tests, it is important to warm up thoroughly.

Stress Test 1

For this test you need a good hill. The hill needs to take you about two minutes to run up it and of sufficient gradient to ensure you are breathing hard at its summit. The test begins around five minutes running time from the hill. Gradually accelerate towards the hill achieving 85% MHR (for the first time) at the base of the hill. As you hit the hill, maintain your speed by increasing your effort. Your heart rate will rise and you will tire. Without falling over, keep an eye on your monitor and make a mental note of your highest heart rate as you work towards the top of the hill.

Stress Test 2

For those unfortunate enough to live in an area lacking hills it is possible to carry out a test on a flat piece of road or at your local running track. The plan of attack is to run 800 meters very quick. For the first 400 meters run at up to your current 90 to 95% MHR (to be achieved by the end of the first lap) and for the last 400 metres go for it. During this second lap, you must work at 100%. Very fit athletes may have to repeat this test after a few minutes rest (minimum of 65% MHR) to be able to achieve a true maximum. This test is very reliable.

Notes

A stress test should be carried out every six months to ensure ongoing accuracy of your training zones. Many athletes do not achieve their actual MHR at the first attempt as they are either not fit enough or are running tired.

It is worth noting you will have different maximum heart rates for different endurance sports, such as cycling. This is due to the number and size of the muscle groups used. Running uses the largest muscle groups in the body and therefore has the highest heart rates associated to it. Cyclists will need to carry out a maximum stress test for that sport to obtain their cycling maximum.

Having determined your maximum heart rate it is now possible to calculate your heart rate training zones.

129

Hip Flexion Test

Testing and measurement are the means of collecting information upon which subsequent performance evaluations and decisions are made but in the analysis we need to bear in mind the factors that may influence the results.

Objective

The objective of this test is to monitor the development of the athlete's hip flexors (the muscles that lift your knees).

Required Resources

To undertake this test you will require:

Non slip surface

How to conduct the test

The athlete lies on their back

The athlete lifts the left knee and using their hands pulls the left knee to their chest.

Normal flexibility is indicated when their right leg remains flat on the floor.

Hip flexors are considered tight if, as they attempt to lift their left knee toward their chest, their right leg leaves the floor.

Repeat with your other leg.

Analysis

Analysis of the result is by comparing it with the results of previous tests. It is expected that, with appropriate training between each test, the analysis would indicate an improvement.

130

Static Flexibility Test - Hip and Trunk

Testing and measurement are the means of collecting information upon which subsequent performance evaluations and decisions are made but in the analysis we need to bear in mind the factors that may influence the results.

Objective

The objective of this test is to monitor the development of the athlete's hip and trunk flexibility.

How to conduct the test

Starting position Sit on the floor with the back and head against a wall, legs fully extended with the bottom of the feet against the sit-and-reach box Place the hands on top of each other, stretching the arms forward while keeping the head and back against the wall Measure the distance from the fingertips to the box edge with a ruler. This becomes zero or starting point

Movement Slowly bend and reach forward as far as possible sliding the fingers along the ruler Hold the final position for two seconds Record the distance reached to the nearest 1/10 of an inch Repeat the test 3 times and note the best distance.

<table>
<tr>
<td>

Starting position

Sit on the floor with the back and head against a wall, legs fully extended with the bottom of the feet against the sit-and-reach box

Place the hands on top of each other, stretching the arms forward while keeping the head and back against the wall

Measure the distance from the fingertips to the box edge with a ruler. This becomes zero or starting point

</td>
<td>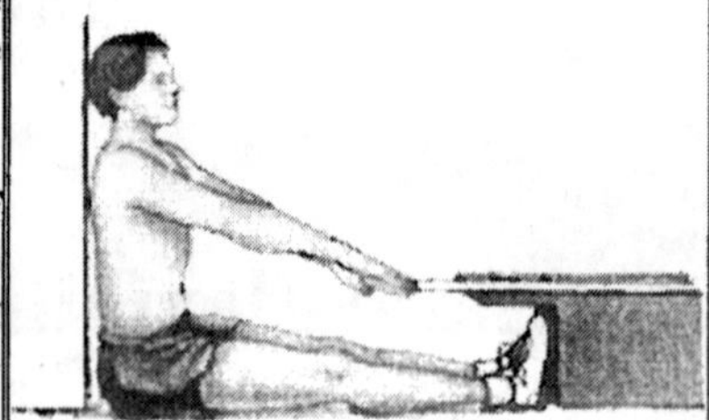</td>
</tr>
<tr>
<td>

Movement

Slowly bend and reach forward as far as possible sliding the fingers along the ruler

Hold the final position for two seconds

Record the distance reached to the nearest 1/10 of an inch

Repeat the test 3 times and note the best distance

</td>
<td>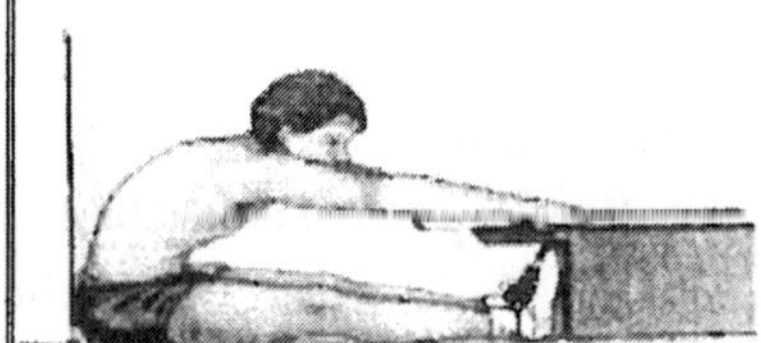</td>
</tr>
</table>

Fig. 48 : Static Flexibility

Analysis

Analysis of the result is by comparing it with the results of previous tests. It is expected that, with appropriate training between each test, the analysis would indicate an improvement.

Fig. 42 : Normative data for the Hip and Trunk flexibility test

Age<36

Rating	*Men*	*Women*
Excellent	>17.9	>17.9
Good	17.0 - 17.9	16.7 - 17.9
Average	15.8 - 16.9	16.2 - 16.6
Fair	15.0 - 15.7	15.8 - 16.1
Poor	<15.0	<15.8

Age 36 to 49

Rating	*Men*	*Women*
Excellent	>16.1	>17.4
Good	14.6 - 16.1	16.2 - 17.4
Average	13.9 - 14.5	15.2 - 16.1
Fair	13.4 - 13.8	14.5 - 15.1
Poor	<13.4	<14.5

Tables adapted from Johnson B.L. & Nelson J.K. Practical Measurements for Evaluation in PE 4th Ed. 1986.

131

Illinois Agility Run Test

Testing and measurement are the means of collecting information upon which subsequent performance evaluations and decisions are made but in the analysis we need to bear in mind the factors that may influence the results.

Objective

The objective of the Illinois Agility Run Test is to monitor the development of the athlete's agility

Required Resources

To undertake this test you will require:

flat surface - a 400 metre Track

8 cones

Stop watch

Assistant

The Illinois course

The length of the course is 10 metres and the width (distance between the start and finish points) is 5 metres. On an athletics track, you could use 5 lanes.

4 cones can be used to mark the start, finish and the two turning points. Each cone in the centre is spaced 3.3 metres apart.

How to conduct the test

The Illinois Agility Run Test is conducted as follows:

The athlete lies face down on the floor at the start point

On the assistant's command the athlete jumps to his/her feet and negotiates the course around the cones to the finish

The assistant records the total time taken from their command to the athlete completing the course.

Analysis

Analysis of the result is by comparing it with the results of previous tests. It is expected that, with appropriate training between each test, the analysis would indicate an improvement.

The following are national norms for 16 to 19 year olds.

Table 43 : Normative data for the Illinois Agility Run Test

Gender	*Excellent*	*Above Average*	*Average*	*Below Average*	*Poor*
Male	<15.2 secs	15.2 - 16.1 secs	16.2 - 18.1 secs	18.2 - 18.3 secs	>18.3 secs
Female	<17.0 secs	17.0 - 17.9 secs	18.0 - 21.7 secs	21.8 - 23.0 secs	>23.0 secs

Table Reference: Davis B. et al; Physical Education and the Study of Sport; 2000.

Target Group

This test is suitable for team sports but not for individuals where the test would be contraindicated.

Reliability

Reliability would depend upon how strict the test is conducted and the individual's level of motivation to perform the test.

Validity

There are published tables to relate results to a potential level of fitness and the correlation is high.

132

Dynamic Knee Extension Test

Testing and measurement are the means of collecting information upon which subsequent performance evaluations and decisions are made but in the analysis we need to bear in mind the factors that may influence the results.

Objective

The objective of this test is to assess the strength of the athlete's knee extensor muscles.

Required Resources

To undertake this test you will require:

Universal knee flexor/extensor bench

Assistant

How to conduct the test

The athlete sits on the end of the bench with the padded edge of the bench against the posterior surface of the knee joint

The feet are hooked behind the padded rollers. The hands grasp the sides of the bench just behind their buttocks

The correct technique involves a complete extension of the knee, conducted in a smooth and continuous movement

The initial resistance should be approximately 33% of male body mass and 25% of female body mass

If the athlete can successfully complete one repetition, repeat the procedure after one minute, adding an additional weight to the previous resistance.

Continue with this procedure, allowing one minute recovery between attempts until the 1RM has been determined

Record the final resistance

Analysis

Analysis of the result is by comparing it with the results of previous tests. It is expected that, with appropriate training between each test, the analysis would indicate an improvement.

133

Kosmin Test

Testing and measurement are the means of collecting information upon which subsequent performance evaluations and decisions are made but in the analysis we need to bear in mind the factors that may influence the results.

Objectives

The Kosmin Test was devised in the USSR to predict an athlete's 800 metre or 1500 metre time.

Required Resources

To undertake this test you will require:

400 metre track

Stop watch

An assistant

How to conduct the test

800 metres

The athlete is required to run two controlled maximal efforts of 60 seconds with a recovery of 3 minutes. The athlete commences their second run from the point where the first run was completed. The total distance covered by the two runs is recorded 1500 metres.

The athlete is required to run four controlled maximal efforts of 60 seconds with a diminishing recovery of 3 minutes, 2 minutes and 1 minute. The athlete commences their next run from the point where the previous run was completed. The total distance covered by the four runs is recorded.

Kosmin Tables

Due to their size, the Kosmin tables have not been included here. However, the athlete's potential 800 metre or 1500 metre time can be predicted by using the Total Distance covered in the following appropriate equation.

Table 44 : Kosmin Table

Gender	*Distance*	*Equation*
Male	800 metres	Time=217.77778 - (Total Distance x 0.119556)
Female	800 metres	Time=1451.46 - (198.54 x Log (Total Distance))
Male	1500 metres	Time=500.52609 - (Total Distance x 0.162174)
Female	1500 metres	Time=(500.52609 - (Total Distance x 0.162174)) + 10

The Kosmin Tables could be created by using these equations in a spreadsheet package e.g. Microsoft Excel.

Analysis

Analysis of the result is by comparing it with the results of previous tests. It is expected that, with appropriate training between each test, the analysis would indicate an improvement.

Target Group

This test is suitable for middle distance athletes but not for individuals where the test would be contraindicated.

Reliability

Reliability would depend upon how strict the test is conducted and the individual's level of motivation to perform the test.

Validity

There are published tables to relate results to potential performance in competition and the correlation is high.

Limitations

The equations can be used for male and female athletes but they do tend to over predict for female athletes. The on line calculators here have taken adjustments for female athletes into consideration.

When to use

To predict performance and monitor progress the Kosmin tests can be used at the:

- beginning of the winter training to establish a baseline (September/October)
- just prior to indoor racing (December/January)
- just prior to thc outdoor season (March/April)

134

LAS Test

Testing and measurement are the means of collecting information upon which subsequent performance evaluations and decisions are made but in the analysis we need to bear in mind the factors that may influence the results.

The LAS (Lactic vs Speed) test, a speed endurance assessment for 400 metre athletes, has been provided by Les Archer - a coach from New Zealand.

Objective

The objective of this test is to monitor the 400 metre athlete's speed endurance.

Required Resources

To undertake this test you will require:

- 400 metre track
- Stop watch
- An assistant

How to conduct the test

- Have the athlete perform a 500 metre time trial
- Record the time (T1)

At least 48 hours later have the athlete perform the following sprints:

- 50 metres - record the time (T2)
- 4 minutes recovery
- 100 metres - record the time (T3)
- 4 minutes recovery
- 150 metres - record the time (T4)
- 4 minutes recovery
- 200 metres - record the time (T5)

Analysis

Sum the times S1 = T2 + T3 + T4 + T5

Compare the times T1 (time for the 500 metre run) and S1 (total time for the sprints) - In my experience the difference should not exceed 5 seconds. If the difference is more than 5 seconds then this indicates a lack of endurance and a difference less than 5 seconds indicates a lack of speed.

Why? This is just a test that I have been using with my athletes for the past 8 years with some great success. Three men have run the 400 metres below 45 seconds and one woman has done sub 51 seconds on this formula. This is not an exact science, but merely a tool to help you.

Analysis of the result is by comparing it with the results of previous tests. It is expected that, with appropriate training between each test, the analysis would indicate an improvement.

135

Lateral Change of Direction Test

Testing and measurement are the means of collecting information upon which subsequent performance evaluations and decisions are made but in the analysis we need to bear in mind the factors that may influence the results.

Objective

To monitor the development of the athlete's speed with directional change.

Required Resources

To undertake this test you will require

- Flat surface - track
- Three cones
- Stop watch
- Assistant

How to conduct the test

The three cones are set five metres apart on a straight line.

The athlete starts at the middle cone.

The Coach gives the signal to start and points in a specific direction, right or left.

The athlete moves to and touches the first cone, returns past the middle cone (start) to the far cone and touches that one and then returns to the middle cone, touching that one.

The coach starts the stopwatch on giving the 'Go' command and stops the watch when the athlete touches the middle cone. The better of the two trails in each starting direction, right and left, are recorded and the best score in each direction is used for scoring.

Analysis

Analysis of the result is by comparing it with the results of previous tests. It is expected that, with appropriate training between each test, the analysis would indicate an improvement.

Normative data for the lateral change of direction test

The following data has been obtained from the results of tests conducted with world class athletes.

Table 45 : Normative Data for the lateral Change of direction test

% Rank	*Females*	*Males*
91-100	-3.22 - 3.37 secs	2.90 - 3.05 secs
81 - 90	3.38 - 3.53 secs	3.06 3.21 secs
71 - 80	3.54 - 3.69 secs	3.22 - 3.37 secs
61 - 70	3.70 - 3.85 secs	3.38 - 3.53 secs
51 - 60	3.86 - 4.01 secs	3.54 - 3.69 secs
41 - 50	4.02 - 4.17 secs	3.70 - 3.85 secs
31 - 40	4.18 - 4.33 secs	3.86 - 4.01 secs
21 - 30	4.34 - 4.49 secs	4.02 - 4.17 secs
11 - 20	4.50 - 4.65 secs	4.18 - 4.33 secs
1 - 10	4.66 - 4.81 secs	4.34 - 4.49 secs

Table reference: D.A. Chu; Explosive Power and Strength; Human Kinetics; 1996.

136

Margaria Kalamen Power Test

Testing and measurement are the means of collecting information upon which subsequent performance evaluations and decisions are made but in the analysis we need to bear in mind the factors that may influence the results.

Objective

The objective of this test is to monitor the development of the athlete's power.

Required Resources

To undertake this test you will require:

Stopwatch

Assistant

Flight of 12 steps with a starting line of 6 metres in front of the first step - each step is about 17.5 cm high with the 3rd, 6th and 9th step brightly coloured.

How to conduct the test

The athlete's weight is determined (kg) and recorded.

The vertical distance between the 3rd and 9th step is recorded.

The athlete undertakes 2 or 3 practice runs up the steps to warm up.

The athlete stands ready at the starting line. On the command "Go", the athlete sprints to the steps and up the flight of steps taking three steps at a time (3rd, 6th and 9th stairs).

Assistant records the time to get from the 3rd step to the 9th step - the stopwatch is to be started with foot contact on the 3rd step and stopped with foot contact on the 9th step.

Athlete repeats the test 2 more times - allow a 2-3 minute recovery between each test.

Analysis

Analysis of the result is by comparing it with the results of previous tests. It is expected that, with appropriate training between each test, the analysis would indicate an improvement.

Power (Watts) is calculated from the formula:

P=(M x D) x 9.8/t where

P = Power (Watts)

M = Body mass (kg)

D = Vertical distance (m)**

t = Time (s)

**The vertical distance (D) between the 3rd and 9th step must be accurately measured and used when calculating the power.

137

McCloy Physical Fitness Test

Testing and measurement are the means of collecting information upon which subsequent performance evaluations and decisions are made but in the analysis we need to bear in mind the factors that may influence the results.

Objective

To monitor the development of the athlete's strength.

Required Resources

To undertake this test you will require:

Gym with mats and a bar on which to do pull ups

Stop watch

Assistant

How to conduct the test

The athlete undertakes a series of exercises with the coach recording the number of repetitions completed for each exercise. The coach should allow a three minute recovery between each exercise. The test comprises of the following exercises:

Chins (Pull Ups) to maximum

Press Ups to maximum
Squat Thrusts for 1 minute
Squat Jumps for 1 minute
Sit Ups for 2 minutes

Analysis

Analysis of the result is by comparing it with the results of previous tests. It is expected that, with appropriate training between each test, the analysis would indicate an improvement.

The Physical Fitness Index (P.F.I.) is calculated by adding together the repetitions completed for each exercise and then dividing the total by five.

138

Muscle Fibre Test

Testing and measurement are the means of collecting information upon which subsequent performance evaluations and decisions are made but in the analysis we need to bear in mind the factors that may influence the results.

Objective

The objective of the muscle fibre test is to determine the fibre composition of the muscles used for a particular exercise. Two test protocols are described: The Dr F. Hatield muscle fibre test and the Charles Poliquin muscle fibre test.

Required Resources

To undertake this test you will require:

Weight training facilities

An assistant/spotter

Selection of exercises

How to conduct the Dr F. Hatfield muscle fibre test

Determine your one repetition maximum (1RM) on an exercise

Rest for 15 minutes

Perform as many repetitions as possible with 80% of your 1RM

Analysis

Less than 7 repetitions - fast twitch (FT) dominant

7 or 8 repetitions - mixed fibre type

more than 8 repetitions - slow twitch (ST) dominant

If you are FT dominant, then you should use heavier loads and lower repetitions predominantly in your training. ST dominant individuals, on the other hand, will respond better to lighter loads and higher repetitions

How to conduct the Charles Poliquin muscle fibre test

Determine your one repetition maximum (1RM) on an exercise Rest for 15 minutes

Perform as many repetitions as possible with 85% of your 1RM

Analysis

Less than 5 repetitions - fast twitch (FT) dominant

5 repetitions - mixed fibre type

more than 5 repetitions - slow twitch (ST) dominant

If you are FT dominant, then you should use heavier loads and lower repetitions predominantly in your training. ST dominant individuals, on the other hand, will respond better to lighter loads and higher repetitions.

139

Modified Sit and Reach Test

Testing and measurement are the means of collecting information upon which subsequent performance evaluations and decisions are made but in the analysis we need to bear in mind the factors that may influence the results.

Objective

The objective of this test is to monitor the development of the athlete's hip and trunk flexibility.

Required Resources

To undertake this test you will require:

A 'sit & reach table'

Yard stick

An assistant

Analysis

Analysis of the result is by comparing it with the results of previous tests. It is expected that, with appropriate training between each test, the analysis would indicate an improvement.

How to conduct the test

Starting position. Sit on the floor with the back and head against a wall, legs fully extended with the bottom of the feet against the sit-and-reach box Place the hands on top of each other, stretching the arms forward while keeping the head and back against the wall Measure the distance from the fingertips to the box edge with a ruler. This becomes zero or starting point	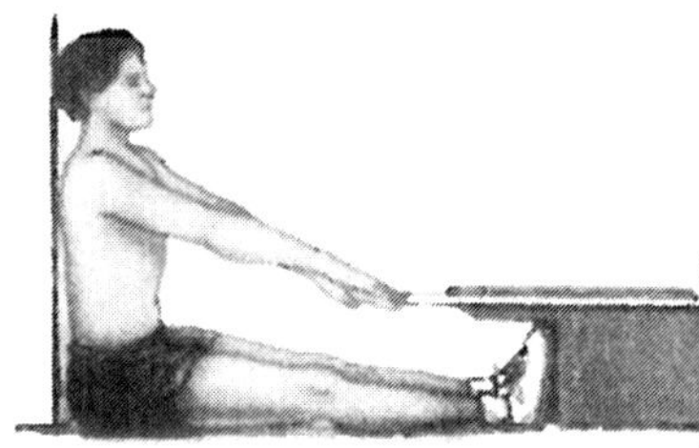
Movement Slowly bend and reach forward as far as possible sliding the fingers along the ruler Hold the final position for two seconds Record the distance reached to the nearest 1/10 of an inch Repeat the test 3 times and note the best distance	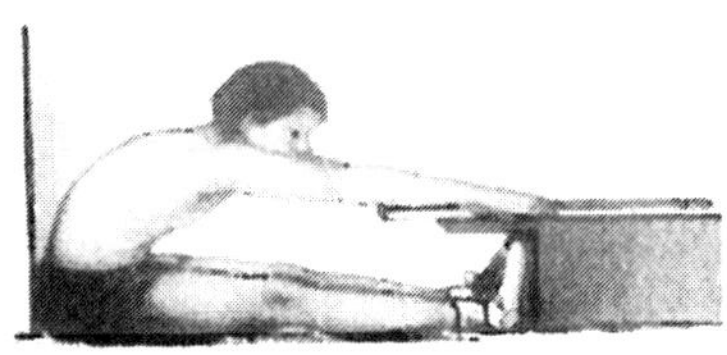

Fig. 49 : Modified Sit and Reach

140

Static Flexibility Test - Trunk and Neck

Testing and measurement are the means of collecting information upon which subsequent performance evaluations and decisions are made but in the analysis we need to bear in mind the factors that may influence the results.

Objective

The objective of this test is to monitor the development of the athlete's trunk and neck flexibility

Starting position

Lay prone on the floor with hands clasped at the side of the head

Movement

Raise the trunk as high as possible whilst keeping the hips in contact with the ground

An assistant can hold the feet down

Record the vertical distance, to the nearest 1/4 of an inch, from the tip of the nose to the ground

Repeat the test 3 times and record the best distance

How to conduct the test

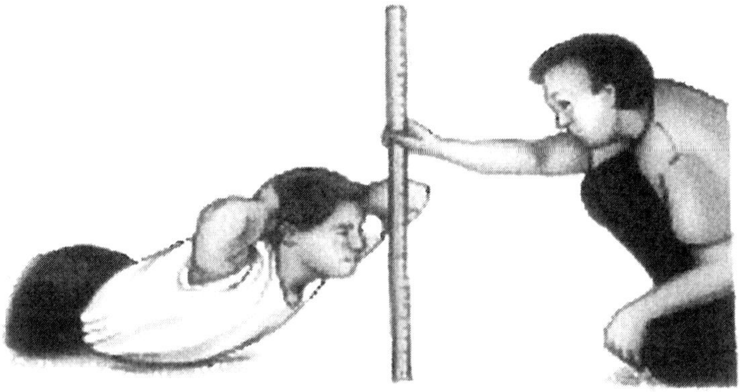

Fig. 50

Analysis

Analysis of the result is by comparing it with the results of previous tests. It is expected that, with appropriate training between each test, the analysis would indicate an improvement.

Table 46 : Normative data for the Trunk and Neck flexibility test

Rating	*Men*	*Women*
Excellent	>10.00	>9.75
Good	10.00 - 8.00	9.75 - 7.75
Average	7.99 - 6.00	7.74 - 5.75
Fair	5.99 - 3.00	5.74 - 2.00
Poor	<3.00	<2.00

Table adapted from Johnson B.L. & Nelson J.K. Practical Measurements for Evaluation in PE 4th Ed. 1986

141

Orthostatic Heart Rate Test

Athletes are often under a lot of pressure to perform well on a regular basis. This pressure can result in the athlete overtraining and/or becoming stressed. The Orthostatic Heart Rate Test is used to monitor the athlete's state of health.

Requirements for the Orthostatic Heart Rate Test

To perform the Orthostatic Heart Rate Test you require

Stop watch

Knowledge of how to take you pulse rate

Performing the Orthostatic Heart Rate Test

- lay down and rest for at least 15 minutes
- record your pulse rate (beats/min) - R1
- stand up
- 15 seconds later record you pulse rate (beats/minute) - R2
- record the difference between R1 and R2

If the difference is greater than 15 to 20 beats then it is probable that the athlete has not recovered from the previous days training or is under stress. The athlete should consider adjusting the training programme to allow them to recover.

Overhead Press Test

Testing and measurement are the means of collecting information upon which subsequent performance evaluations and decisions are made but in the analysis we need to bear in mind the factors that may influence the results.

Objective

The objective of this test is to monitor the strength of the athletes elbow extensors and superior shoulder girdle muscles.

Required Resources

To undertake this test you will require:

- Universal overhead press station
- A supportive lumbar lifting belt
- Assistant

How to conduct the test

- A supportive lumbar lifting belt is recommended for this exercise during maximal lifts
- The athlete stands and leans into the apparatus with the back leg straight and the front foot leg bent at the knee at about 150 degrees
- The hand grips are adjacent to the front of the shoulders
- The initial resistance should be about 33% of male body mass and 25% of female body mass
- As the weight is lifted, the body should move slightly forward so that the extended arms and trunk and rear leg should form a straight line
- If the athlete can successfully complete one repetition, repeat the procedure after one minute, adding an additional weight to the previous resistance
- Continue with this procedure, allowing one minute recovery between attempts until the 1RM has been determined
- Record the final resistance

Analysis

Analysis of the result is by comparing it with the results of previous tests. It is expected that, with appropriate training between each test, the analysis would indicate an improvement.

Target Group

This test is suitable for active athletes but not for individuals where the test would be contraindicated.

142

Press Up Test

Testing and measurement are the means of collecting information upon which subsequent performance evaluations and decisions are made but in the analysis we need to bear in mind the factors that may influence the results.

Objective

The objective of the Press Up test is to assess the endurance of the athlete's upper body muscles.

Required Resources

To undertake this test you will require:

- flat surface
- mat
- a partner

How to conduct the test

The Press Up Test is conducted as follows: Lie on the mat, hands shoulder width apart and fully extend the arms - see Fig. 51 Lower the body until the elbows reach 90° - see Fig. 51 Return to the starting position with the arms fully extended - see Fig. 51 The feet are not to be held The push up action is to be continuous with no rest Complete as many push ups as possible Record the total number of full body press ups.

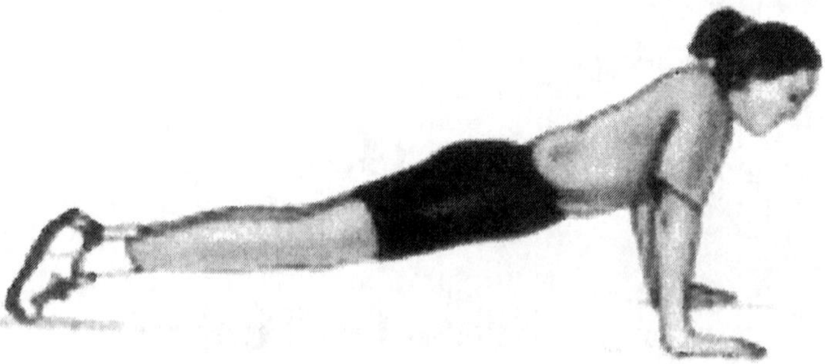

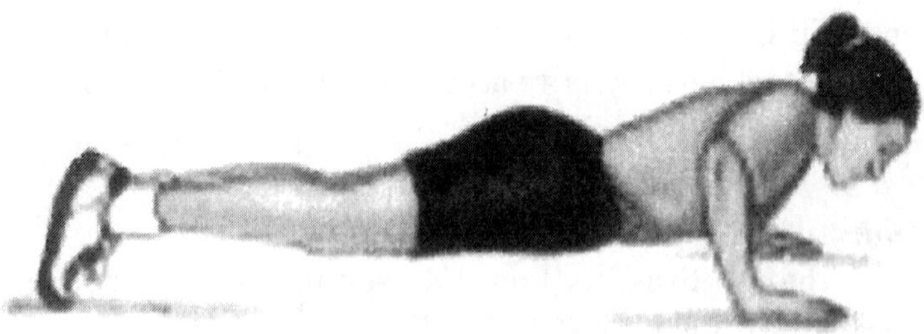

Fig. 51 : Press Up

Female athletes tend to have less relative strength in the upper body and therefore can use the modified press up position to assess their upper body strength. The test is then performed as follows: Lie on the mat, hands shoulder width apart, bent knee position and fully extend the arms - see Fig. 51 Lower the upper body until the elbows reach 90° - see Fig. 51 Return to the starting position with the arms fully extended - see Fig. 51 The feet are not to be held The push up action is to be continuous with no rest Complete as many modified push ups as possible Record the total number of modified press ups.

Table 47 : Normative data for the Press Up Tests

Full body press up

Age	*Excellent*	*Good*	*Average*	*Fair*	*Poor*
20 - 29	>54	45 - 54	35 - 44	20 - 34	<20
30 - 39	>44	35 - 44	25 - 34	15 - 24	<15
40 -49	>39	30 - 39	20 - 29	12 - 19	<12
50 - 59	>34	25 - 34	15 - 24	8 - 14	<8
60+	>29	20 - 29	10 - 19	5 - 9	<5

Modified Push Ups

Age	*Excellent*	*Good*	*Average*	*Fair*	*Poor*
20 - 29	>48	34 - 38	17 - 33	6 - 16	<6
30 - 39	>39	25 - 39	12 - 24	4 - 11	<4
40 -49	>34	20 - 34	8 - 19	3 - 7	<3
50 - 59	>29	15 - 29	6 - 14	2 - 5	<2
60+	>19	5 - 19	3 - 4	1- 2	<1

Table Reference: McArdle W.D. et al; Essential of Exercise Physiology; 2000

Target Group

This test is suitable for active individuals but not for those where the test would be contraindicated.

Reliability

Reliability would depend upon, how strict the test is conducted and the individual's level of motivation to perform the test.

143

Ruler Drop Test

Testing and measurement are the means of collecting information upon which subsequent performance evaluations and decisions are made but in the analysis we need to bear in mind the factors that may influence the results.

Objective

The objective of this test is to monitor the athlete's reaction time.

Required Resources

To undertake this test you will require.

- A one 1 metre ruler
- An assistant

How to conduct the test

The ruler is held by the assistant between the outstretched index finger and thumb of the athlete's dominant hand, so that the top of the athlete's thumb is level with the zero centimetre line on the ruler. The assistant instructs the athlete to catch the ruler as soon as possible after it has been released.

The assistant is to record distance between the bottom of the ruler and the top of the athlete's thumb where the ruler has been caught.

Analysis

The algorithm to calculate the reaction speed is **$d = vt + ½at^2$** where

- d = distance in metres
- v = initial velocity = 0
- a = acceleration due to gravity = $9.81 m/s^2$
- t = time in seconds

We need to manipulate **$d = vt + ½at^2$** to give us an algorithm for **t**

As **v** = 0 then **vt** = 0 therefore the algorithm is **t = Sqrt (2d/a)**

Example

- d = 9cm
- t = sqrt(2 × 0.09 ÷ 9.81)
- t = sqrt(0.01835)
- t = 0.135 seconds

Analysis of the result is by comparing it with the results of previous tests. It is expected that, with appropriate training between each test, the analysis would indicate an improvement.

Table 48 : Normative data for the Ruler Drop Test

The following are national norms for 16 to 19 year olds.

Excellent	*Above Average*	*Average*	*Below Average*	*Poor*
<7.5cm	7.5 - 15.9cm	15.9 - 20.4cm	20.4 - 28cm	>28cm

Table Reference: Davis B. et al; Physical Education and the Study of Sport; 2000

Target Group

This test is suitable for all athletes but not for individuals where the test would be contraindicated.

Reliability

Reliability would depend upon, how strict the test is conducted and the individual's level of motivation to perform the test.

Validity

There are no published tables to relate results to potential performance in competition.

144

Rast

Testing and measurement are the means of collecting information upon which subsequent performance evaluations and decisions are made but in the analysis we need to bear in mind the factors that may influence the results.

Objective

The Running-based Anaerobic Sprint Test (**RAST**) was developed at the University of Wolverhampton (United Kingdom) to test an athletc's anaerobic performance. RAST is similar to the Wingate ANaerobic 30 cycle Test (WANT) in that it provides coaches with measurements of power and fatigue index. The Wingate test is more specific for cyclists whereas the RAST provides a test that can be used with athletes where running forms the basis of the movement.

Required Resources

To undertake this test you will require:

400 metre track - with a 35 metre marked section on the straight

Two cones to mark the 35 metre section

Stop watch

An assistant

How to conduct the test

The athlete :

is weighed prior to the test

undertakes a 10 minute warm session

has a 5 minute recovery

completes six 35 metre runs at maximum pace (10 seconds allowed between each sprint for turnaround)

The assistant

records the time taken for each 35 metre sprint to the nearest hundredth of a second

makes appropriate calculations

Analysis

Analysis of the result is by comparing it with the results of previous tests. It is expected that, with appropriate training between each test, the analysis would indicate an improvement.

Calculations

Power output for each sprint is found using the following equations

- Velocity = Distance ÷ Time

Acceleration = Velocity ÷ Time

Force = Weight × Acceleration

Power = Force × Velocity

OR

Power = Weight × Distance ^{2} ÷ Time ^{3}

From the six times calculate the power for each run and then determine :

Maximum power - the highest value

Minimum power - the lowest value

Average power - sum of all six values ÷ 6

Fatigue Index - (Maximum power - Minimum power) ÷ Total time for the 6 sprints

Example

Athlete weight = 76 Kilograms

Sprint	*Time (secs)*	*Power (watts)*
1	4.52	1008
2	4.75	869
3	4.92	782
4	5.21	658
5	5.46	572
6	5.62	525

Interpretation of the results

Maximum Power

Is a measure of the highest power output and provides information about strength and maximal sprint speed. Research range is 1054 watts to 676 watts.

Minimum Power

Is the lowest power output achieved and is used to calculate the Fatigue Index. Research range is 674 watts to 319 watts.

Average Power

Gives an indication of an athlete's ability to maintain power over time. The higher the score the better the athlete's ability to maintain anaerobic performance.

Fatigue Index

Indicates the rate at which power declines for the athlete. The lower the value the higher the ability for the athlete to maintain anaerobic performance. With a high fatigue index value (>10) the athlete may need to focus on improving their lactate tolerance.

How to use

The test is conducted on a regular basis throughout the training program. Results should be compared with the athlete's previous results to determine if the training program is achieving the desired results. Results can then be used to appropriately adjust the athlete's training program.

When to use

RAST can be used on a regular basis (3 to 6 weeks) throughout the season. The period between tests will be determined by the training phase and the amount of training being conducted.

Target Group

This test is suitable for sprint and endurance athletes and players of endurance sports (e.g. football, rugby) but not for individuals where the test would be contraindicated.

Reliability

Reliability would depend upon, how strict the test is conducted and the individual's level of motivation to perform the test.

Validity

There are no published tables to relate results to potential performance in competition.

145

Exercise Intensity and Energy Source

Energy is primarily supplied from two sources:

Carbohydrates - in the form of glycogen stored in the muscles

Fat - stored around the body

During exercise, we use a combination of these energy sources. At a high intensity the main source of energy is carbohydrate and at a low intensity, fat is the predominate source. As there is a limit to the amount of carbohydrate that can be stored in the muscles, high intensity work can only be sustained for short periods. We have large stores of fat so low intensity work can be maintained for long periods.

Exercise Intensity and Energy Source

The relationship between exercise intensity (% of your Maximum Heart Rate) and the energy source (carbohydrate and fat) is as follows:

Table 49 : Exercise Intensity and Energy

Intensity % MHR	*% Carbohydrate*	*% Fat*
65 to 70	40	60
70 to 75	50	50
75 to 80	65	35
80 to 85	80	20
85 to 90	90	10
90 to 95	95	5
100	100	0

146

Respiratory Exchange Ratio (RER)

Carbohydrates, fat and protein all play a part in energy metabolism and for a certain volume of oxygen the energy released will depend upon the energy source. It is possible to estimate which particular fuel (carbohydrate, fat or protein) is being oxidised by calculating the Respiratory Exchange Ratio (RER). RER is the ratio of carbon dioxide (CO_2) produced to oxygen (O_2) consumed and is known as the Respiratory Quotient (RQ).

If carbohydrate is completely oxidised to CO_2 and water (H_2O) then the relationships is as follows:

$6O_2 + C_6H_{12}O_6$ » $6CO_2 + 6H_2O + 38ATP$ (Adenosine Triphosphate)

$RER = 6CO_2 \div 6O_2 = 1$

If fat (e.g. palmitic acid) is completely oxidised to CO_2 and H_2O then the relationships is as follows:

$C_{16}h_{32} + 23O_2$ » $16CO_2 + 16H_2O + 129ATP$

$RER = 16CO_2 \div 23O_2 = 0.7$

The RER for protein is approx. 0.8 but as it plays a very small part in energy metabolism, it is not important here. A value between

0.7 and 1.0 indicates a mixture of fat and carbohydrate as the energy source. A value greater than 1.0 indicates anaerobic respiration due to more CO2 being produced than 02 consumed.

147

Resting Daily Energy Expenditure

Using your weight, height and age it is possible to determine your resting daily energy expenditure (RDEE). This method was validated in 1919 by Dr. J.A. Harris and Dr. F.G. Benedict using closed circuit spirometry.

Concept 2 Rowing Step Test

Testing and measurement are the means of collecting information upon which subsequent performance evaluations and decisions are made but in the analysis we need to bear in mind the factors that may influence the results.

Objective

To monitor the development of the athlete's anaerobic throshold.

Required Resources

To undertake this test you will require:

Concept 2 Rowing Machine

Heart rate monitor

An assistant

How to conduct the test

The test consists of five four minute rows, each rowed at a constant 500 metre pace. The pace is increased for each step and you have a 30 second recovery between each row. Use the calculator below to determine the pace for each step. The 5th step is at 100% (maximum) effort.

For each step, you need to record the set 500 metre/pace, distance rowed in 4 minutes, the stroke rate, the actual 500 metre pace and steady state heart rate. Heart rate reaches its steady state after approximately 3 minutes of rowing.

Analysis

Analysis of the results is by comparing it with the results of previous tests. Improvement in endurance is indicated when you find that the steady state heart rate is lower for any given 500 metre pace when compared to a previous test. It is expected that, with appropriate training between each test, the analysis would indicate an improvement in the athlete's anaerobic threshold.

Example

The following is an example of a test for an athlete whose best time for the 2000 metres is 6 minutes and 32 seconds, which is an average 500 metres split of 1 minute 38 seconds.

Step 1 - 4 minutes at 1 minute 59 seconds/500 metres

30 seconds recovery - record distance, stroke rate, set & actual 500 metres pace and steady pace heart rate

Step 2 - 4 minutes at 1 minute 54 seconds/500 metres

30 seconds recovery - record distance, stroke rate, set & actual 500 metres pace and steady pace heart rate

Step 3 - 4 minutes at 1 minute 50 seconds/500 metres

30 seconds recovery - record distance, stroke rate, set & actual 500 metres pace and steady pace heart rate

Step 4 - 4 minutes at 1 minute 47 seconds/500 metres

30 seconds recovery - record distance, stroke rate, set & actual 500 metres pace and steady pace heart rate

Step 5 - 4 minutes at Maximum effort

Record distance, stroke rate, actual 500 metres pace and steady pace heart rate

148

Scat

By analysing an athlete's responses to a series of statements about how she/he feels in a competitive situation it is possible to determine their level of anxiety. A test that provides such functionality is the Sport Competition Anxiety Test (SCAT) that was developed by Martens, Vealcy, and Burton in 1990.

Assessing Your Anxiety

Read each statement below, decide if you "Rarely", "Sometimes" or "Often" feel this way when competing in your sport, select the appropriate radio button to indicate your response and then select the "Analyse" button to see your test result.

Do not spend too long on each statement, as there is no right or wrong answers. Your SCAT score will range from a low of 10 to a high of 30 where 10 indicates a low level of anxiety and 30 a high level of anxiety (stressed).

Competing against others is socially enjoyable

Before I compete I feel uneasy

Before I compete I worry about not performing well

I am a good sportsman when I compete

When I compete, I worry about making mistakes

Before I compete I am calm

Setting a goal is important when competing

Before I compete I get a queasy feeling in my stomach

Just before competing, I notice my heart beats faster than usual

I like to compete in games that demands a lot of physical energy

Before I compete I feel relaxed

Before I compete I am nervous

Team sports are more exciting than individual sports

I get nervous wanting to start the game

Top of Form

Before I compete I usually get uptight

149

Squats Test

Testing and measurement are the means of collecting information upon which subsequent performance evaluations and decisions are made but in the analysis we need to bear in mind the factors that may influence the results.

Objective

The objective of this test is to monitor the development of the athlete's leg strength

Required Resources

To undertake this test you will require:

A chair that makes your knees bend at right angles when you are sitting

Assistant

How to conduct the test

Stand in front of a chair, facing away from it, with your feet shoulders width apart

Squat down and lightly touch the chair with your backside before standing back up

Keep doing this until you are fatigued

Record the number of squats completed

Analysis

Analysis of the result is by comparing it with the results of previous tests. It is expected that, with appropriate training between each test, the analysis would indicate an improvement.

Table 50 : Normative Data for Squat Tests

Male

Age	*18-25*	*26-35*	*36-45*	*46-55*	*56-65*	*65+*
Excellent	>49	>45	>41	>35	>31	>28
Good	44-49	40-45	35-41	29-35	25-31	22-28
Above average	39-43	35-39	30-34	25-38	21-24	19-21
Average	35-38	31-34	27-29	22-24	17-20	15-18
Below Average	31-34	29-30	23-26	18-21	13-16	11-14
Poor	25-30	22-28	17-22	13-17	9-12	7-10
Very Poor	<25	<22	<17	<9	<9	<7

Female

Age	*18-25*	*26-35*	*36-45*	*46-55*	*56-65*	*65+*
Excellent	>43	>39	>33	>27	>24	>23
Good	37-43	33-39	27-33	22-27	18-24	17-23
Above average	33-36	29-32	23-26	18-21	13-17	14-16
Average	29-32	25-28	19-22	14-17	10-12	11-13
Below Average	25-28	21-24	15-18	10-13	7-9	5-10
Poor	18-24	13-20	7-14	5-9	3-6	2-4
Very Poor	<18	<20	<7	<5	<3	<2

Target Group

This test is suitable for active athletes but not for individuals where the test would be contraindicated.

Reliability

Reliability would depend upon, how strict the test is conducted and the individual's level of motivation to perform the test.

Validity

There are no published tables to relate results to potential performance in competition.

150

Static Flexibility Test - Shoulder and Wrist

Testing and measurement are the means of collecting information upon which subsequent performance evaluations and decisions are made but in the analysis we need to bear in mind the factors that may influence the results.

Objective

The objective of this test is to monitor the development of the athlete's shoulder and wrist flexibility.

How to conduct the test

Starting Position	
• Lay prone on the floor with the arms fully extended holding a stick	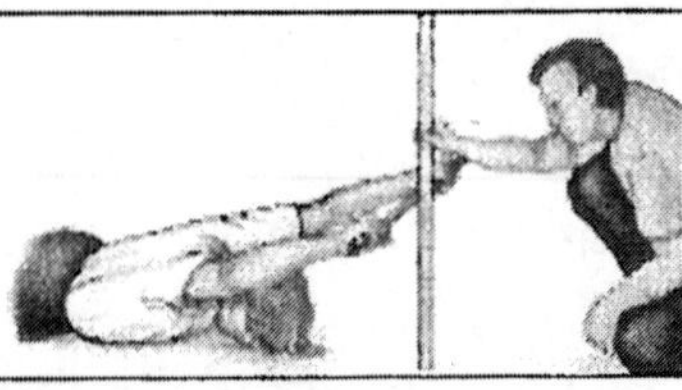

Fig. 52 : Static Flexibility

Movement

- Raise the stick as high as possible, keeping the nose on the ground
- Measure the vertical distance the stick rises from the floor to the nearest 1/2 inch
- Repeat the test 3 times and record the best distance
- Measure the arm length from the acromial extremity to the tip of the longest finger

Subtract the best score from the arm length

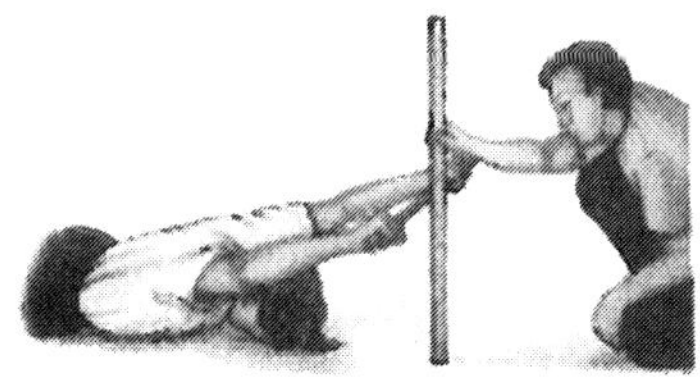

Fig. 53 : Static Flexibility

Table 51 : Normative data for the Shoulder and Wrist flexibility test

Rating	*Men*	*Women*
Excellent	>12.50	>11.75
Good	12.50 - 11.50	11.75 - 10.75
Average	11.49 - 8.25	10.74 - 7.50
Fair	8.24 - 6.00	7.49 - 5.50
Poor	<6.0	<5.50

Table adapted from Johnson B.L. & Nelson J.K. Practical Measurements for Evaluation in PE 4th Ed. 1986.

Analysis

Analysis of the result is by comparing it with the results of previous tests. It is expected that, with appropriate training between each test, the analysis would indicate an improvement.

151

Static Flexibility Test - Shoulder

Testing and measurement are the means of collecting information upon which subsequent performance evaluations and decisions are made but in the analysis we need to bear in mind the factors that may influence the results.

Objective

The objective of this test is to monitor the development of the athlete's shoulder flexibility.

How to conduct the test

Starting position

- Grasp one end of the rope with the left hand
- Four inches away grasp the rope with the right hand

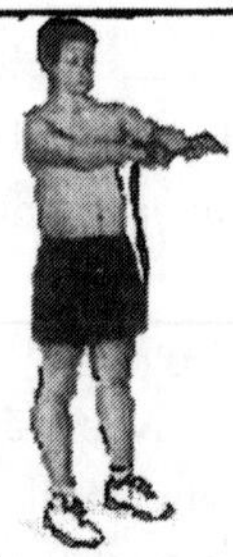

Fig. 54 : Static Flexibility

Movement

- Extend both arms in front of the chest and rotate the arms overhead and behind the neck until the rope touches the back
- As resistance occurs allow the right hand to slide along the rope
- Measure the distance between the two thumbs - to the nearest 1/4 of an inch
- Measure shoulder width from deltoid to deltoid - to the nearest 1/4 of an inch
- Subtract the shoulder width distance from the thumb distance

Repeat the test 3 times and record the best distance

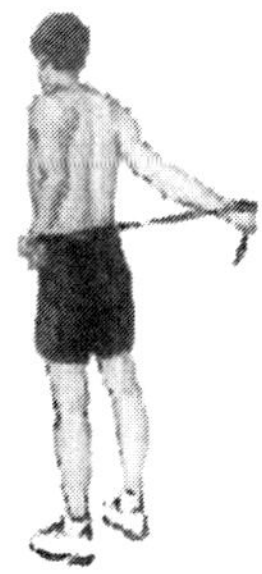

Fig. 55 : Static Flexibility

Analysis

Analysis of the result is by comparing it with the results of previous tests. It is expected that, with appropriate training between each test, the analysis would indicate an improvement.

Table 52 : Normative data for the Shoulder flexibility test

Rating	*Men*	*Women*
Excellent	<7.00	<5.00
Good	11.50 - 7.00	9.75 - 5.00
Average	14.50 - 11.49	13.00 - 9.74
Fair	19.75 - 14.49	17.75 - 12.99
Poor	>19.75	>17.75

Table adapted from Johnson B.L. & Nelson J.K. Practical Measurements for Evaluation in PE 4th Ed. 1986.

152

'T' Drill Test

Testing and measurement are the means of collecting information upon which subsequent performance evaluations and decisions are made but in the analysis we need to bear in mind the factors that may influence the results.

Objective

To monitor the development of the athlete's speed with directional change.

Required Resources

To undertake this test you will require:

- Flat surface
- Four cones
- A stop watch
- An assistant

How to Conduct the Test

Three cones are set five metres apart on a straight line. A fourth cone is placed 10 metres from the middle cone so that the cones form a 'T'.

- The athlete starts at the cone at the base of the 'T'
- The coach gives the signal to 'Go' and starts the stop watch
- The athlete runs to the middle cone, touches the cone

- The athlete then side steps 5 metres to the left cone, touches that cone
- The athlete then side steps 10 metres to the far cone and touches that one
- The athlete the side steps 5 metres back to the middle cone, touching that one
- The athlete then runs 10 metres backwards to the base of the 'T' and touches that cone
- The coach stops the watch

153

Tecumseh Step Test

Testing and measurement are the means of collecting information upon which subsequent performance evaluations and decisions are made but in the analysis we need to bear in mind the factors that may influence the results.

Objective

The objective of this test is to monitor the development of the athlete's cardio respiratory fitness.

Required Resources

To undertake this test you will require:

A gym bench or step (8 inches/20.3 cm high)
A stop watch
An Assistant

How to Conduct the Test

The Tecumseh Step Test is conducted as follows:

- Perform a step cycle of four-step cadence (right foot up, left foot up, right foot down and left foot down) completing 24 cycles in one minute. This is 2 cycles in a 5 second period.
- Have someone to help you keep to the required pace or you could use a metronome set at 96 beats/minute.

- Perform the test for 3 minutes
- 30 seconds after finishing the test count the number of pulse beats for 30 seconds

The number of beats counted in 30 seconds is then used in the table below to determine the athlete's grade.

154

VO2 Max Step Test

Testing and measurement are the means of collecting information upon which subsequent performance evaluations and decisions are made but in the analysis we need to bear in mind the factors that may influence the results.

Objective

The objective of this test is to monitor the development of the athlete's cardiovascular system.

Required Resources

To undertake this test you will require:

- A 16¼ inch high bench or step
- A stop watch
- Metronome or cadence tape
- Heart rate monitor (optional)
- An assistant

How to conduct the test

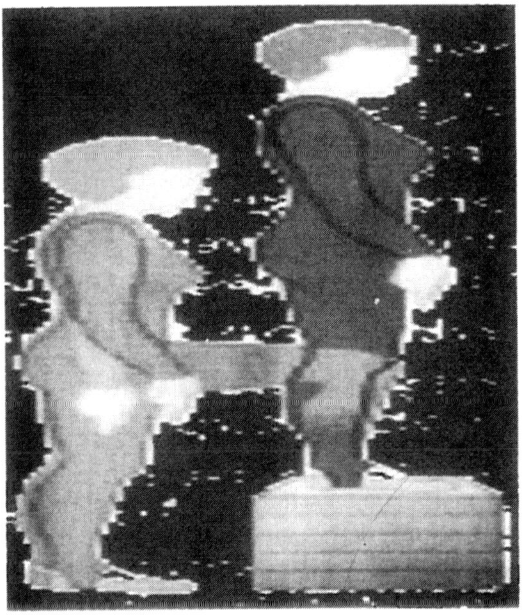

Fig. 56 : Step Test

The VO2 max Step Test is conducted as follows:

- Step up and down, one foot at a time, onto the step or bench for 3 minutes
- Maintain a steady four beat cycle
    - Women 22 steps/minute
    - Men 24 steps/minute
- On finishing the test count the number of heart beats for 15 seconds
- Multiply the number of beats in 15 seconds by 4 to give the "step test pulse rate"
- Use this final value to assess the athlete's VO2 max using the calculator below

Analysis

Analysis of the result is by comparing it with the results of previous tests. It is expected that, with appropriate training between each test, the analysis would indicate an improvement.

155

Wall Squat Test

Testing and measurement are the means of collecting information upon which subsequent performance evaluations and decisions are made but in the analysis we need to bear in mind the factors that may influence the results.

Objective

To monitor the development of the athlete's quadriceps strength endurance.

Required Resources

To undertake this test you will require:

- Warm dry location – gym
- Smooth wall
- Stop watch
- An assistant

How to conduct the test

- Stand comfortable on both feet with your back against a smooth wall
- Slide your back down the wall to assume the position shown in the diagram

- There is to be a 90° angle at the hip and knee

When you are ready

- Lift one foot 5 cm off the ground
- Assistant starts the stop watch
- Balance for as long as possible
- The watch is stopped when you put your foot back on the ground

Take a rest and then repeat the test with the other leg.

Table 53 : Normative data for the Wall Squat Test

The following are national norms for 16 to 19 year olds.

Gender	*Excellent*	*Above Average*	*Average*	*Below Average*	*Poor*
Male	>102 secs	102 – 76 secs	75 – 58 secs	57 – 30 secs	<30 secs
Female	>60 secs	60 – 46 secs	45 – 36 secs	35 – 20 secs	<20 secs

Table Reference: Arnot R and Gaines C, Sports Talent, 1984

156

Wheelchair VO2max Test

Testing and measurement are the means of collecting information upon which subsequent performance evaluations and decisions are made but in the analysis we need to bear in mind the factors that may influence the results.

Objective

To monitor the athlete's level of aerobic fitness.

Required Resources

To undertake this test you will require:

400 metre track – marked every 100 metres

Stop watch

Assistant

How to Conduct the Test

The test comprises of seeing how far an athlete can travel in twelve minutes. The assistant should record the total distance covered to the nearest 100 metres.

Analysis

Analysis of the result is by comparing it with the results of previous tests. It is expected that, with appropriate training between each test, the analysis would indicate an improvement.

References

1. Advanced PE for Edexcel, F. Galligan et al., ISBN 0 435 506439
2. Advanced Studies in Physical Education and Sport, P Beashel et al., ISBN 0 17 4482345
3. Armstrong, L.E. (2000). Performing in Extreme Environments, Human Kinetics, Champaign, IL.
4. Armstrong, L.E., Maresh, C.M., Castellani, J.W., Bereron, M.F., Kenefick, R.W., LaGassee, K.E., and Riebe, D. (1994). "Urinary Indices of Hydration Status.", Int. J. Sport Nutr., 4, 265-279.
5. Armstrong, L.E., Soto, J.A., Hacker, F.T., Casa, D.J., Kavouras, S.A., Maresh, C.M. (1998). "Urinary indices during dehydration, exercise, and rehydration." Int. J. Sport Nutr. 8: 345-355.
6. Astrand Treadmill VO2max Calculator - a free Microsoft Excel spread sheet that you can download and use on your computer.
7. Bailey, D.A., R.J. Shephard and R.L. Mirwald. Validation of a self-administered home test of cardiorespiratory fitness. *Can. J. Appl. Sport Sci.* 1: 67-78, 1976.
8. Borg, G, "Perceived Exertion as an indicator of somatic stress", Scandinavian journal of Rehabilitation Medicine 1970, 2(2), 92-98
9. Bosco C, Luhtanen P, Komi PV (1983) *A simple method for measurement of mechanical power in jumping*. **European Journal of Applied Physiology** 50:273-282.
10. Bouchard, C. and R.J. Shephard. A new approach to the interpretation of Canadian Home Fitness Test scores. *Can. J. Sport Sci.* In Press, 1993.

11. Brouha L, Health CW, Graybiel A. *Step test simple method of measuring physical fitness for hard muscular work in adult men.* **Rev Canadian Biol**, 1943 ;2:86
12. Burmeister, W (1965), *Potassium-40 Content as a Basis for the Calculation of Body Cell Mass in Man.* Science 148, 1336-1337.
13. Cooper, K.H. (1968) A means of assessing maximal oxygen uptake. Journal of the American Medical Association 203:201-204.
14. Davis B. et al; Physical Education and the Study of Sport; 2000
15. Davis OM. *Exercise capacity of individuals with paraplegia.* Med Sci Sports Exerc 1993;25(4):423-32.
16. Dawson, B., Ackland, T., Roberts, C., & Lawrence, S (1991) *Repeated effort testing:The phosphate recovery test revisited.* **Sports Coach** 14(2): 12-17
17. Dawson, B.; Ackland, T.; Roberts, C. Kirby, R.F. (1991). *Phosphate Recovery Test [Power Test of the Legs / Lower Body - Running Test].* (1984). IN: **Kirby's guide to fitness and motor performance tests.** BenOak Pub. Co. Cape Girardeau, MO. Page(s): 370-371.
18. Essentials of Exercise Physiology, W.D. McArdle et al., ISBN 0 683 30507 7
19. Examining Physical Education, K. Bizley, ISBN 0 435 50660 9
20. Fitness Canada. *Canadian Standardized Test of Fitness (CSTF) Operations Manual.* 3rd Ed. Ottawa: Fitness and Amateur Sport, Canada, 1986.
21. Franklin BA, Swantek KI, Grais SL, Johnstone KS, Gordon S, Timmis GC. *Field test estimation of maximal oxygen consumption in wheelchair users.* Arch Phys Med Rehabil 1990;71(8):574-78.
22. Gilbert B. Forbes, James Gallup, and John B. Hursh, (1961) *Estimation of Total Body Fat from Potassium-40 Content,* Science 13, Vol. 133. no. 3446, pp.101-102.
23. Hanson, P. (1984) *Clinical Exercise Training.* In: **Sport Medicine**. Ed: Strauss, R. Philadelphia, PA: W.B. Saunders Company. 13-40.

24. Hartung GH, LaHy DA, Blaneq RJ. *Comparison of treadmill exercise testing protocols for wheelchair users.* Eur J Appi Physiol Occup Physiol 1993;66(4):362-65.

25. *International Standards for Anthropometric Assessment* (2001) published by The International Society for the Advancement of Kinanthropometry (ISAK)

26. J P Buckley, J Sim, R G Eston, R Hession, R Fox, *Reliability and validity of measures taken during the Chester step test to predict aerobic power and to prescribe aerobic exercise.* **Br J Sports Med** 2004;38:197–205.

27. Jetté, M., J. Campbell, J. Mongeon and R. Routhier. The Canadian Home Fitness Test as a predictor of aerobic capacity. *Can. Med. Assoc.* J. 114: 680-682, 1976

28. Johnson BL, Nelson JK. Practical measurements for evaluation in physical education. 4th Edit. Minneapolis: Burgess, 1979.

29. Kalamen, J. (1968) *Measurement of maximum muscular power in man.* Doctoral thesis, Ohio State University

30. KEEN EN, SLOAN AW. *Observations on the Harvard step test.* **J Appl Physiol.** 1958 Sep;13(2):241-3.

31. Krustrup, P., Mohr, M., Amstrup, T., Rysgaard, T., Johansen, J., Steensberg, A.,Redersen, P, K., Bangsbo, J. (2003) *The Yo-Yo Intermittent Recovery Test:Physiological Response, Reliability, and Validity.* Medicine & Science in Sports & Exercise. 35(4), 697-705.

32. L.A. & Lambert, J. (1982) "A maximal multistage 20m shuttle run test to predict VO2 max", European Journal of Applied Physiology, Vol 49, p1-5.

33. Leger, L.A. & Lambert, J. (1982) "A maximal multistage 20m shuttle run test to predict VO2 max", European Journal of Applied Physiology, Vol 49, p1-5.Leger,

34. *Marc Vanderthommen, Marc Francaux, Cédrik Colinet, Cédric Lehance, Claude Lhermerout, Jean-Michel Crielaard, Daniel Theisen, A multistage field test of wheelchair users for evaluation of fitness and prediction of peak oxygen consumption*, Journal of Rehabilitation Research and Development, Dec 2002, Volume:39 Issue:6 Page:685-692.

35. Margaria, R., Aghemo, P. and Rovelli, E. (1966) Measurement of muscular power (anaerobic) in man. *Journal of Applied Physiology* 221, 1662-1664.
36. Meyers CR., *A study of the reliability of the Harvard step test.* **Res Q**. 1969 May; 40(2): 423.
37. Minikin, B., 1990, Hints for interpreting the Tri-level profile of general fitness, in Sports Coach, Vol.13, No. 3, p21.
38. Montoye HJ, Willis PW 3rd, Cunningham DA, Keller JB. *Heart rate response to a modified Harvard step test: males and females, age 10-69.* **Res Q.** 1969 Mar;40(1):153-62.
39. MONTOYE HJ. *The Harvard step test and work capacity.* **Rev Can Biol.** 1953 Mar;11(5):491-9.
40. PE for you, J. Honeybourne, ISBN 0 7487 3277 2
41. Physical Education and Sport Studies, D. Roscoe et al., ISBN 1 901424 20 0
42. Physical Education and the Study of Sport, B. Davis et al., ISBN 0 7234 31752
43. Physiology Matters, David M Wilkinson (1999).
44. Rechichi, C. Dawson, B. & Lawrence, S.R. (2000). *A multistage shuttle swim test to assess aerobic fitness in competitive water polo players.* Journal of Science and Medicine in Sport. 3(1): 55-64.
45. REEDY JD, SAIGER GL, HOSLER RH. *Evaluation of the Harvard Step Test with respect to factors of height and weight.* **Int Z Angew Physiol**. 1958;17(2):115-9.
46. Rhodes EC, McKenzie DC, Coutts KD, Rodgers AR. *A field test for the prediction of aerobic capacity in the male paraplegics and quadraplegics.* Can J Appl Sport Sci 1981;6(4):182-86.
47. Ricci B, Baldwin K, Hakes R, Fein J, Sadowsky D, Tufts S, Wells C., *Energy cost and efficiency of Harvard step-test performance.* **Int Z Angew Physiol.** 1966 Apr 28;22(2):125-30.
48. Rosin, R and Shulov, A (1961), *Estimation of total body fat from potassium-40 content.* Science, 133, 1918.
49. RYHMING I. *A modified Harvard step test for the evaluation of physical fitness.* **Arbeitsphysiologie**. 1953;15(3):235-50.

50. Sayers, S., et al. (1999) *Cross-validation of three jump power equations.* **Med Sci Sports Exerc.** 31: 572.
51. Shephard, R.J. Current status of the Canadian Home Fitness Test. *Br. J. Sports Med.* 14: 114-125, 1980.
52. Shephard, R.J. *Fitness of a Nation. Lessons from the Canada Fitness Survey.* Basel: S. Karger A.G., 1986.
53. Shephard, R.J., S. Thomas and I. Weller. The Canadian Home Fitness Test. 1991 Update. *Sports Medicine* 11: 358-366, 1991.
54. Sloan AW., *A modified Harvard step test for women.* **J Appl Physiol.** 1959 Nov;14:985-6.
55. Sport and PE, K Wesson et al., ISBN 0 340 683821
56. summarised from the Eurofit for adults book: Assessment of Health Related Fitness, Council of Europe Publishing.
57. Sykes K and Roberts A, *The Chester step test—a simple yet effective tool for the prediction of aerobic capacity,* **Physiotherapy,** Volume 90, Issue 4, December 2004, Pages 183-188.
58. Sykes K. Chester step test; resource pack (Version 3). Cheshire, UK: Chester College of Higher Education, 1998.
59. Telford, R.D., Minikin, B.R., Hahn, A.G., & Hooper, L.A., 1989. A simple method for the assessment of general fitness: The Tri-level profile. Australian Journal of Science and Medicine in Sport, 21 (3): p. 6-9.
60. The World of Sport Examined, P. Beashel et al., ISBN 0 17 438719 9
61. Vanlandewijck YC, Daly DJ, Theisen DM, *Field test evaluation of aerobic anaerobic, and wheelchair basketball skill performances.* Int J Sports Med 1990;20(8):548-54.
62. Vinet A, Bernard PL, Poulain M, Varray A, Le Gallais D, Micallcf JP, *Validation of an incremental field test for the direct assessment of peak oxygen uptake in wheelchair dependent athletes.* Spinal Cord 1996;34(5):288- 93.

Index